Thomas Platz, Cosima Pinkowski

Frederike van Wijck, Garth Johnson

# ARM – Arm Rehabilitation Measurement

Thomas Platz, Cosima Pinkowski
Frederike van Wijck, Garth Johnson

# ARM – Arm Rehabilitation Measurement

Manual for performance and scoring of the

*Fugl-Meyer test (arm section),*

*Action Research Arm test,* and the

*Box-and-Block test*

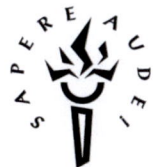

Deutscher Wissenschafts-Verlag (DWV)

Baden-Baden

**Autoren:**

**Priv.-Doz. Dr.med. Thomas Platz**
Arzt für Neurologie, Rehabilitationswesen
Dipl. in Epidemiology and Biostatistics
(Mc Gill)
Charité – Universitätsmedizin Berlin
Campus Benjamin Franklin
Abteilung für neurologische Rehabilitation
Klinik Berlin
Kladower Damm 223
D–14089 Berlin

**Frederike van Wijck, MSc BSc MCSP ILTM**
Lecturer
School of Health Sciences
Queen Margaret University College
Leith Campus
Duke Street
UK–Edinburgh EH6 8HF

**Dipl. Med.-Päd. Cosima Pinkowski**
Ergotherapeutin
HAWK, Hochschule für Angewandte
Wissenschaft und Kunst
Fachhochschule Hildesheim / Holzminden /
Göttingen
Fakultät Soziale Arbeit und Gesundheit
Tappenstraße 55
D–31134 Hildesheim

**Professor Garth R Johnson, PhD FREng**
Centre for Rehabilitation and Engineering
Studies
School of Mechanical & Systems Engineering
University of Newcastle upon Tyne
Stephenson Building
Claremont Road
UK–Newcastle upon Tyne NE1 7RU

**Cover-Gestaltung:** Priv.-Doz. Dr.med. Thomas Platz

**Bibliografische Information Der Deutschen Bibliothek**
Die Deutsche Bibliothek verzeichnet diese Publikation in der
Deutschen Nationalbibliografie; detaillierte bibliografische
Daten sind im Internet über http://dnb.ddb.de abrufbar.

1. Auflage
Gedruckt auf alterungsbeständigem, chlorfrei gebleichtem Papier

© Copyright 2005 by
Deutscher Wissenschafts-Verlag (DWV)®
Postfach 11 01 35
D–76487 Baden-Baden

www.dwv-net.de

ISBN: 3-935176-42-2

# Preface

Rehabilitation, like medicine in general, is changing rapidly. In the last years new therapeutic regimes, new training devices and pharmacologic approaches were introduced, often however without a sound evaluation of these methods. Traditional methods in rehabilitation are also often lacking a scientific basis.

Therefore, due to scares resources, the efficacy and cost-effectiveness of interventions is more and more questioned and has to be demonstrated. This trend for evidence based rehabilitation necessitates the use and evaluation of proper outcome measures.

In contrast to general activities of daily living (ADLs) or to spasticity, motor assessment of arm functions is still not done in clinical routine. Either the clinicians lack the information or the training to use proper scales in this field.

The present book "ARM – Arm Rehabilitation Measurement" written by Dr. Platz and co-authors gives an excellent overview and presents a very practical manual for three commonly used assessment tools: the Fugl-Meyer Test, the Action Research Arm Test (ARAT) and the Box and Block Test.

First it characterizes the individual test, points out the theories and ideas behind, gives a concise description of the performance and of the test properties. Since detailed user manuals are not available for many motor assessment scores a very useful and detailed manual was developed for the three mentioned tests. Starting positions, detailed instructions to the patient, scoring guidelines are provided (and were developed during the DRAMA Project (Developments in Rehabilitation of the Arm) sponsored by the European Commission).

The manual is a very suitable means to enable standardisation and to assure reliable and repeatable results in different institutions. The book is very well written and attractively illustrated.

Therefore I would wish for the book a broad audience in order to improve the outcome assessment and in the end the therapeutic effectiveness of neurological rehabilitation.

Professor Karl-Heinz Mauritz
Regional European Vice President
World Federation of Neurorehabilitation

*Berlin, March 2005*

# Table of contents

# 1. Overview

There are significant numbers of people with neurological disabilities throughout the world, the most common problems being stroke (CVA), multiple sclerosis (MS) and traumatic brain injury (TBI). The majority of these people suffer from a loss of arm function, which often affects their independence and increases their need for health care services. Thus, loss of arm function in CVA, MS and TBI constitutes a major socio-economic burden on communities.

To establish the efficacy and cost-effectiveness of intervention, outcome assessment is crucial. However, the latter is not done routinely or in a standardised way. One of the main reasons for this appears to be a lack of information and training regarding the application of clinical rating scales and in particular, measurement technology to the assessment of motor deficits in neurological rehabilitation. There is a need for comprehensive and appropriate resources for effective teaching and learning with respect to this important subject.

This book, dedicated to assessment of the upper limb in neurological rehabilitation, was designed to support those who want to assess arm function in patients with neurodisabilities, especially as caused by arm paresis.

## 2. Introduction

There are significant numbers of people with neurological disabilities throughout the world, the most common problems being stroke (CVA), multiple sclerosis (MS) and traumatic brain injury (TBI). Due to the nature of the lesion(s) in the central nervous system, the majority of these people suffer from a loss of arm function. This often affects their independence and increases their need for health care services, such as physiotherapy, occupational therapy and various forms of care in the community. Thus, in addition to affecting the quality of life of those affected by their disability (as well as their carers), loss of arm function in CVA, MS and TBI constitutes a major socio-economic burden on communities. Furthermore, since the proportion of elderly people with neurological impairments is growing, this burden is increasing.

In rehabilitation, long and short term goals are set to demarcate the path towards optimum levels of functioning. For patient, clinician and funding body involved in this process, it is important to monitor the achievement of these goals as well as the cost-effectiveness of the management process itself. There is mounting pressure on clinicians to document clinical outcomes routinely and to provide evidence of treatment efficacy. Clinical scales of arm function can be used to diagnose, quantify and monitor functional deficits in terms of impairment (e.g. degree of paresis) and activity limitations (e.g. ADL) (WHO, 2001).

Standardised assessment of functional status and outcome is a central component of both clinical practice and research. In clinical practice, standardised outcome assessment is one of the cornerstones of total quality management (Whetsell, 1995; Epstein, 1995). In clinical research, standardised motor assessment can be used to evaluate the efficacy of treatment methods such as training strategies or medication (e.g. Langhammer and Stanghelle, 2000; Miltner et al., 1999; Platz et al., 2001; Platz et al., in press [a]; Walker-Batson et al., 1995). Further, it is a prerequisite for the investigation of modifiers of motor recovery, e.g. the role of psychological variables or brain activation patterns in motor recovery (Nelles et al., 2001; Platz et al., 2002; Platz and Denzler, 2002; Platz et al., in press [b]).

Despite the published data on motor assessment scales (for review see Wade, 1992) and their potential for outcome monitoring, they are not widely used in routine neurological rehabilitation. In order to identify current patterns in the usage of clinical scales and measurement technology for the assessment of motor deficits in neurological rehabilitation, a survey was carried out in the context of this project (van Wijck et al. 2001). The results showed that clinical rating scales are not used routinely or in a standardised way. Generally, respondents indicated that the centres where they are based use a number of different clinical assessment scales (median 3), most frequently with a small proportion of patients. The (Modified) Ashworth Scale, the Functional Independence Measure and the Fugl-Meyer are used most frequently. Just over half the number of respondents stated that their centre used one or more scales in more than 75% of their patients, but the choice of such routinely used instruments varies widely, indicating poor standardisation between centres. The lack of quantification and standardisation of the assessment of motor deficits involving the upper limb in neurological patients seriously impairs the development of evidence based practice. It emerged from the survey that there is a clear need for information and training regarding the usage of clinical rating scales.

There are a number of reasons for the low frequency of scale usage. Importantly, there appears to be a lack of information and training on how to use these scales (van Wijck et al, 2001).

In general, users rely on original publications for reference, which focus on psychometric properties rather than provide the necessary detailed guidance for performance and scoring of the test. Consequently, users must specify their own test criteria to achieve a high degree of standardisation. This is certainly possible as has been proven by successful single centre reliability studies (e.g. Duncan et al., 1983; Hsieh et al., 1998; Sanford et al., 1993; van der Lee et al., 2001).

Manuals specifically addressing issues of performance and scoring of motor scales have the advantage of promoting standardisation and allowing communication and comparison of research results across clinical centres, which is a prerequisite for conducting multi-centre trials.

One aim of a project named DRAMA (Developments in Rehabilitation of the Arm) sponsored by the European commission was, to develop and evaluate standardised assessment manuals for selected clinical tools. The Department of Neurological Rehabilitation at the Charité – Universitäts-medizin Berlin, Germany, acted as Lead Clinical Partner and was in charge of these clinical aspects of the project. The authors of this book developed the manuals. Together with Centro Studi Neurolesi Messina (Italy) and the Centre for Rehabilitation and Engineering Studies at the University of Newcastle upon Tyne (CREST, UK), the training manuals were piloted and clinical data for a multicentre reliability and validity study were collected (Platz et al., 2005) (for details see also chapter 4).

Specifically, a detailed user manual was developed for the Fugl-Meyer test (arm section), the Action Research Arm test, and the Box-and-Block test. The manual- and video-based assessment of patients with arm paresis enabled standardisation of test administration and scoring and thus assured reliable and valid arm motor assessment across facilities and with retesting. The three arm motor tests provide information that is (1) not identical to information provided by a more generic scales of neurological impairment and (2) quite independent of a person's ability to cope with basic activities of daily living.

# 3. Characterisation of arm assessment scales

## 3.1. Fugl-Meyer test

### 3.1.1. Idea and Theories

Fugl-Meyer et al. (1975) designed a method for evaluation of physical performance of post-stroke hemiplegic patients which included findings of Twitchell (1951), Reynolds et al. (1958) and Brunnström (1966). Twitchell stated that if motor recovery after onset of brain damage occurs, this process follows an obligatory path. Brunnström and co-workers observed a regular order of restoration of motor functions among stroke patients (Reynolds et al., 1958; Brunnström, 1966). Based on the idea of consecutive steps of recovery from hemiparesis after stroke, the latter developed an assessment protocol, which was later standardised and modified by Fugl-Meyer and co-workers. Accordingly, this instrument is named the Fugl-Meyer test (synonym: Brunnström-Fugl-Meyer test).

The structure of the measurement method is based on the following assumptions:

- conventional testing of muscle strength is inadequate for evaluating motor function in hemiplegic persons
- disorganisation of complex reflex mechanisms is responsible for the lack of highly selective movements after brain injury
- recovery of motor function takes place in stages
- flaccid paresis often precedes changes in reflexes and these are probably associated with the re-acquisition of voluntary movements
- recovery often starts with movements in proximal joints, while movements in distal joints tend to occur later in the process of recovery
- movement synergies, especially of proximal arm activity, are involved in the recovery process and can be the major basis of active motor function at early to intermediate stages of recovery.


The authors expected that a hemiplegic patient shows recurrence of reflex activities before volitional motor functions occur. „Thereafter, through initial dependence on synergies, the active motion will become successively less dependent upon the primitive reflexes and reactions, and finally complete voluntary motor function with normal muscles reflexes may be regained. As the motor function of the wrist and hand may recover somewhat independently of that of the arm, these functions are tested separately." (Fugl-Meyer et al., 1975, 14)

Thus, the stages were defined as follows:
1) reflexes reoccur
2) stereotyped volitional movements can be initiated within flexor and extensor synergies
3) movements can be performed with little or no synergy dependence
4) reflexes are normalised (Duncan et al., 1983).
According to these ideas, the motor items within the test are organised in a specific order.

Since sensory deficits, limited range of motion and joint pain during movement can all influence motor behaviour, their evaluation is also implemented in the test.

If the above mentioned theoretical considerations are valid, the test - given its corresponding structure - should enable the detection of deficits and changes in motor function throughout the whole process of motor rehabilitation. Evidence regarding the test's validity is summarised in chapter 3.1.5.

### 3.1.2. Description
The Fugl-Meyer test consists of unilateral tasks and movements. The motor tasks are ordered according to presumed stages of recovery; with each motor subtest being composed of 1 to 7 items. The patient is asked to perform single- or multi-joint movements and to maintain a position in another joint, to reach and control a starting position, to grasp objects and to hold them against resistance. Although wrist and hand functions are tested as distinct units without involving the proximal joints, various

starting positions are implemented, i.e. elbow 90° and 180° for the wrist items. Co-ordination and speed for the upper limb are measured by applying the finger-to-nose test and observing dysmetria and tremor as well as time taken to complete the task. The two aspects of sensation (light touch, position sense) are assessed qualitatively. The quality of sensation is compared with the non-affected side.

Each side is evaluated separately.

The sections of the Fugl-Meyer test are:

**Motor function upper extremity**

A    Shoulder/Elbow/Forearm

    I    reflex activities

    II    volitional movement in the dynamic flexor and extensor synergies

    III    volitional motion performed with a mix of the dynamic flexor and the extensor synergies

    IV    volitional movements performed with little or no synergy dependence

    V    normal reflex activity

B    Wrist

C    Hand

D    Co-ordination/Speed

**Motor function lower extremity**

E    Hip/Knee/Ankle

    I    reflex activities

    II    volitional movement in the dynamic flexor and extensor synergies

    III    volitional motion performed with a mix of the dynamic flexor and the extensor synergies

    IV    volitional movements performed with little or no synergy dependence

    V    normal reflex activity

F    Co-ordination/Speed

G    Balance

**H Sensation (both upper and lower limb)**

    a    Light touch

    b    Position sense

**J Passive Joint Motion/Joint pain (both upper and lower limb)**

### 3.1.3. Performance

The patient is seated on a chair without arm rests. Each item is performed as a distinct unit, starting with the less- or non-impaired limb. It is very important for every observation of motor performance to ensure that the patient is well instructed and knows what he or she is required to do. Verbal explanation as well as demonstration are the most common strategies to prevent any misunderstanding. The motor items often require a standardised starting position and control of more than one joint. In addition, there are motor items where the assessor is allowed to support the patient to gain and/or maintain a specific position, while the patient performs a movement in another joint (e.g. supporting the elbow position during the wrist tasks). Any detail is described carefully in chapter 5.2. The assessor should be confident that the patient performs optimally and in a valid manner. It is recommended to ask the patient to perform the task first with the unaffected side. Then the evaluator should correct if necessary. It is not meaningful and, more so, it is impossible to interpret scores for motor behaviour that was not performed strictly according to the task requirements of each item.

Although Fugl-Meyer designed the test in a specific order, it may be meaningful to start with the sections on joint motion and joint pain (section J). Joint pain can affect active motion, thereby masking the best possible motor function. Knowledge of the impairments of passive range of motion will influence the way of scoring the motor items. E.g. a patient who suffers on orthopaedic limitations by shoulder abduction will gain a score of „2", when he/she is able to reach his passive range of motion during the task „flexor synergy". Joint motion and position sense are tested in comparison to the non-affected side. The comparison with the non-affected side is, however, less meaningful in patients with bilateral impairment, i.e. in MS or TBI patients. In these cases, it would be recommended to refer to what might normally be expected as normal passive joint motion or position sense.

The test requires some equipment, which is easily available (see box).

Material for the Fugl-Meyer Test

reflex hammer

pencil

paper sheet

cylindrical object
(e.g. eraser fluid: diameter 3.0 cm)

tennis ball

stopwatch

### 3.1.4. Scoring

The scoring system applies a cumulative numerical score. All items of the Fugl-Meyer Test are scored according to a 3 point ordinal scale, except reflex activities (dichotomous). Generally speaking, the scores represent „no function, partial function and perfect function" with the maximum of 226 points for an un-impaired person. Fugl-Meyer et al. preferred a three point scale since 5 or 7 steps in a scale are more prone to low reliability.

| Maximal points for | Motor function upper extremity | 66 |
| --- | --- | --- |
| | Motor function lower extremity | 34 |
| | Balance | 14 |
| | Position sense | 16 |
| | Exteroception | 8 |
| | Passive joint motion | 44 |
| | Joint pain | 44 |
| | Total score | 226 |
| | | |
| | Total score motor function (A-F) | 100 |
| | Total score sensation | 24 |
| | Total score upper extremity | 106 |
| | Total score lower extremity except balance | 86 |

Whilst scoring is always based on a three-point scale, further specific scoring guidelines exist for each item of the motor part and for each subtest. The scoring guidelines reflect the theoretical assumptions regarding different stages of motor recovery and related motor behaviour. An example is the performance of voluntary abduction in the shoulder joint (active movement without synergy): the patient is instructed to abduct the arm to 90° with the elbow fully extended and the forearm pronated. The important observation for scoring is not only whether the patient abducts or not. Rather, the evaluator focuses on the patient's ability to abduct and simultaneously keep the elbow extended and the forearm pronated. Scoring is dependent on the ability to move without synergy and not just to perform the target movement. Consequently, the patient obtains a score of „0" for any immediate supination and flexion at the elbow while attempting to abduct the arm in the shoulder joint and a score of „1" if supination and/or flexion occur in a later phase of the movement. The patient obtains a score of „2" when he or she is able to abduct the arm up to 90 ° without these specified signs of synergy. Thus, the result combines the range of movement and the dependence on synergy.

For scoring of "pronation and supination of the forearm" items it is important whether starting positions can be obtained and whether pro- and supination can be performed. For scoring of "wrist" items it is important whether the required wrist movements can be performed and whether target positions can be held against gravity or resistance.

The hand section covers a wide range of functions. Starting with „some active flexion" and „release of an active mass flexion grasp" the patient has to use specific types of grasp and to hold objects against gravity or against a sudden tug to obtain the maximum score.

Co-ordination/speed of the upper extremity is judged according to the degree of dysmetria, tremor and time needed while carrying out the Finger-to-Nose test.

The results of the examination can be expressed as percentage of the maximum score. According to percentage of maximal score, Fugl-Meyer et al. distinguished between four stages of recovery.

Later, Fugl-Meyer (1980) suggested to group patients according to various levels of impairment based on the Fugl-Meyer Test motor score with a maximum score of 100 points as follows:

< 50    points          severe motor impairment

50-84  points          marked motor impairment

85-95  points          moderate motor impairment

96-99  points          slight motor impairment

### 3.1.5. Test Properties

Since the Fugl-Meyer Assessment is a widely accepted measurement tool both in research and clinical settings, literature search revealed a considerable number of studies describing test properties. Sanford et al. (1993) described 10 studies published between 1975 and 1990. The main concern of this work was construct validity, data concerning criterion validity and reliability.

#### Reliability

In his follow-up study, Fugl-Meyer et al. (1975) found very small divergences in testing, both in item-by-item and in total scores. These results support the reliability of the assessment, although this was not a formal reliability study. Duncan et al. (1983) investigated test-retest and interrater reliability for several subtests, in a group of 18 chronic hemiplegic patients (time after onset between 15 and 99 months) with various levels of impairment. Test-retest reliability was shown to be extremely high. Interrater reliability was high, although the number of patients was limited and one rater misunderstood the scoring guidelines for upper extremity reflexes and co-ordination. It may be possible that aphasia and comprehension deficits reduce the test-retest reliability. Sanford et al. (1993) again demonstrated high reliability coefficients. Analysis of variance results with the components „subject, rater, occasion" led to a high overall reliability (ICC=0.96). Except pain (ICC=0.61), all coefficients were above 0.85, upper extremity ICC=0.97. The authors stated that the Fugl-Meyer assessment is a moderately reliable tool.

A separate analysis of the sensory scale indicated that both the interrater reliability and the internal consistency of the Fugl-Meyer sensation scores were excellent (ICC=0.93, Cronbach's alpha at four time points ranging from 0.94 to 0.98); the light touch items achieved the lowest interrater reliability coefficients (weighted kappa ranging from 0.30 to 0.55) (Lin et al., 2004).

## Validity

Fugl-Meyer demonstrated the validity by graphically plotting the order of development of the sequential stages of motor return of upper and lower limb. Internal validity has been shown by establishing four stages of recovery. Results of the follow-up study conducted by Fugl-Meyer et al. (1975) supported the internal validity by showing that the stages of recovery proceeded as predicted (Fugl-Meyer et al., 1975; De Weerdt & Harrison, 1985). Due to the wide range of the scale (0 –106 points for the upper extremity), the test may well discriminate among more severely impaired and among milder affected patients. The wide range of points does also support the sensitivity to change of the assessment. Sensitivity to change was also demonstrated to be good by Filiatrault et al. (1991). They investigated the test results of stroke patients in a rehabilitation centre (time after onset: mean 4 months) over a period of two months including three assessments. In stroke patients with severe arm paresis the test was more sensitive to therapeutic change early after stroke than the Action Research Arm Test (Platz et al., in press [a]) while the opposite was true in chronic stroke patients treated for learned non-use (van der Lee et al., 2001).

De Weerdt & Harrison (1985) stated that the test has no ceiling effect because it indicates changes throughout the whole process of rehabilitation. However, a maximum score does not necessarily reflect a non-impaired performance nor full strength.

Concurrent validity was demonstrated by several authors: Fugl-Meyer studied the correlation between motor score and ADL-capacities by applying the test to 60 hemiplegic patients more than one year after disease onset and found a high correlation (0.76 to 0.98) (Fugl-Meyer, 1976a&b).

Significant positive correlations were determined between test results and ADL-capacity (with Barthel Index r=.75 and .85 (Wood-Dauphinee et al., 1990), also findings by Fugl-Meyer & Jääskö, (1980) as well as Lindmark & Hamrin (1988). In contrast to the high correlation coefficients of the

Fugl-Meyer scores with the Barthel Index as revealed by Wood-Dauphinee et al. (1990), Duncan et al. (1992; r=0.80 to 0.91) and Hsueh et al. (2001; r>or=0.78), Filiatrault et al. (1991) demonstrated a moderate relation of rho=0.60. Wood-Dauphinee et al. conducted their study with 172 stroke patients up to 5 weeks after onset (mean age 73.7 years), whereas Filatrault included 18 stroke patients (mean age 52.2 years) with a mean time after onset of 4 months. The indicated difference could probably be explained by the suggestion that chronic stroke patients can regain independence in activities of daily life by compensation techniques without regard to the level of arm function.

In addition, significant positive correlations were found between test results and leisure time activities (Sjögren & Fugl-Meyer, 1982).

Kusoffsky et al. (1982) demonstrated significant correlations between motor function (measured as Fugl-Meyer scores) and somatosensory evoked potentials, by applying both procedures to stroke patients from subacute stage to 6 months after onset. The correlation with the upper extremity scores was the highest.

Feys et al. (2000) investigated the predictive value of the Fugl-Meyer test, upper limb section. They demonstrated that the motor score obtained by the Fugl-Meyer test could explain the largest proportion of the variance when predicting motor recovery at two, six and 12 months.

The upper extremity section covariated closely with the test designed by De Souza (1980a) (Berglund & Fugl-Meyer, 1986). The correlation explained more than 90% of variance; comparing only the motor parts, the correlation explained more than 80% of variance (linear regression coefficient =0.95 and Spearman's rho=0.90).

Concurrent validity was also demonstrated with the Action Research Arm Test: Spearman rho=0.91 (2 weeks after onset) and 0.94 (8 weeks after onset) (De Weerdt & Harrison, 1985) as well as with all components of the Arm Motor Ability Test: r=0.92 to 0.94 (in chronic stroke patients) (Chae et al., 2003). Fugl-Meyer scores were also highly correlated with STREAM scores (Stroke Rehabilitation Assessment of Movement) that measure motor and mobility problems in stroke patients (rho=0.95; Wang et al., 2002). A high correlation between Fugl-Meyer upper limb motor score and hand grip force ratio was found with r=.84 (Boissy et al., 1999). Lin & Sabbahi (1999) presented a high reverse correlation (Spearman rho

-0.83 and -0.76) between Fugl-Meyer wrist score and spasticity as assessed with the modified Ashworth Scale.

Due to the ordinally scaled results no norms are available.

The paragraph might be concluded with a citation from Duncan and co-authors (Duncan et al., 1983, 1609). „The Fugl-Meyer assessment technique is an efficient measurement tool that can be performed in approximately 30 minutes. Using the Fugl-Meyer assessment in conjunction with other assessments (ADL, gait, and perceptual-motor), therapists should be able to plan appropriate treatment programs and measure progress. This assessment is a much needed and apparently sound measurement device for research efforts. With this assessment tool, therapists can begin to make comparative analyses of their treatment techniques, analyse trends in recovery of sensorimotor function, and examine factors that might positively influence recovery."

### 3.1.6. Purpose

Fugl-Meyer designed this instrument for the assessment of recovery of motor function in hemiplegic stroke patients, from very early stages with severe impairment to high levels of recovery. In addition to motor function, he included aspects of sensation, balance, passive joint motion and joint pain during motion, and developed a cumulative numerical scoring system.

Contrary to ADL measures, which reflect not only motor function but also any compensatory mechanisms, this test leads to an adequate, reproducible and fairly standardised picture of a patient's sensorimotor and joint characteristics. However, the score does not in itself imply a detailed therapeutical treatment plan since it only gives a survey of impairment.

For those, who look for an instrument to group their patients, Crow et al. (1989) suggest the following groups:

| | | |
|---|---|---|
| Group 1 | initial score | 0-11 |
| Group 2 | initial score | 12-22 |
| Group 3 | initial score | 23-32 |
| Group 4 | initial score | 33 and over |

### 3.1.7. Comments

The test instructions as provided in the article by Fugl-Meyer et al. (1975) give an overview of the test items and scoring guidelines. Nevertheless, by applying this instrument the necessity for even more precise information in terms of performance and scoring became evident. Since our team had to administer and score the test in a standardised way across countries, it was decided to establish a detailed manual based on the basics of Fugl-Meyer et al., it consists of the original text from Fugl-Meyer et al., supplemented with additional specifications and clarifying comments.

As with most evaluation tools, the assessor is likely to experience difficulties with applying the test in a valid manner when comprehension deficits occur (esp. in the items which assess sensation), when the patient suffers from non-fluent dysphasia or when the patient is not able to co-operate for other reasons.

The test has been developed for assessing motor function and recovery in hemiplegic patients. Any concomitant impairment associated with altered movement capacities such as ataxia, extrapyramidal movement disorders or orthopaedic conditions, may compromise the validity of the assessment or even render a valid assessment impossible.

One of its strengths is that it systematically goes through full range of movement for each of the joints of the upper limb (both PRoM and ARoM) and, by progressively moving from associated to dissociated movement patterns, the Fugl-Meyer test can be used to assess patients at both the lower and higher end of the spectrum of recovery.

Each item includes a description of the guidelines on both performance and scoring procedure (compare chapter 5.2.). It is essential that the assessor undergoes a training period to become familiar with them. If the assessor does not have an in-depth knowledge of the scoring guidelines for each task, it will be difficult to prevent invalid performance (e.g. when the evaluator does not keep in mind that the patient has to maintain elbow extension during shoulder abduction, he may fail to correct the patient and will not obtain information on whether the patient is able to perform as instructed or not).

Despite scalability, no abbreviated form of the test has been established.

## 3.2. Box and Block test

### 3.2.1. Idea and Theories

The Box and Block test (BBT) has been first developed by A. Jean Ayres and Patricia Holser Buehler for evaluating gross manual dexterity when applied to adults with cerebral palsy. Patricia Holser Buehler and Elisabeth Fuchs adapted the original version and created the present form of the box in 1957 (Cromwell, 1976). The test has been used as a measure of gross manual dexterity and as a prevocational test for handicapped persons. Norms had been established for children and for adults with neuromuscular deficits. In 1985, Mathiowetz et al. published slightly modified and standardised instructions and norms for adults. These guidelines were used in almost all more recent publications.

### 3.2.2. Description

The test material consists of two adjacent boxes of the same size, one of them filled with 150 blocks. The size of the blocks is 2.5 cubic cm (1 inch). Between the two boxes there is a partition with a height of 15.2 cm. To avoid the noise produced by falling blocks, it is recommended to put some cushioning material, e.g. felt, on the bottom of the box, both in- and outside.

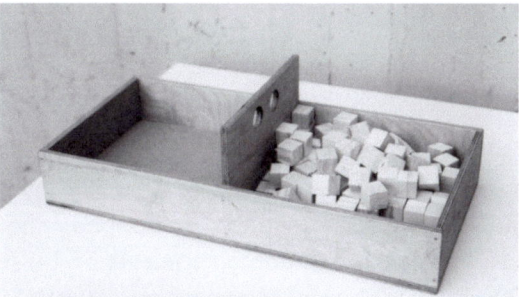

Figure: Box and Block test

The testing equipment is made of 1 cm plywood. The outside dimensions of the long sides are 53.7 x 8.5 cm, the short ends are 25.4 cm long

### 3.2.3. Performance

The performance is based on the guidelines provided by Mathiowetz et al. (1985). A 15 second trial period in advance of the original test is regarded sufficient. They modified the test instruction and designed a standardised procedure for placing the box, for reading the instruction and for scoring.
The blocks are randomly distributed in the field near to the hand which is assessed. The box stands close to and centred in front of the patient.
The patient is well instructed (refer to standardised instruction guidelines in chapter 5.4.) and performs the test first with the less or non-impaired extremity for a 15 second trial. The test trial consists of 60 seconds, where the patient grasps as many blocks as possible, one by one. Each block is brought across with the fingers crossing the partition. After that, the patient releases the block, but it is not necessary to place them on the bottom of the box. The patient is neither asked to take two blocks, nor to pick up blocks which fall outside the box.

### 3.2.4. Scoring

The score is the number of blocks transported from one compartment in the other compartment in one minute thus yielding parametric data. The examiner has to observe whether the performance is valid, since two blocks at a time count for one, whereas a block without the finger tips crossing the partition does not count at all.

### 3.2.5. Test Properties

#### Reliability

Test-retest reliability at six month intervals has been described with rho coefficients of 0.94 (left hand) and 0.98 (right hand) (Cromwell, 1976).
Interrater reliability has been reported by applying this instrument to healthy subjects. Pearson correlation coefficients of 1.0 (right hand) and 0.99 (left hand) were described by Mathiowetz et al. (1985).
Desrosiers et al. (1994) demonstrated a high test-retest reliability by applying the tool to an client group over 60 years (ICC of 0.96 to 0.97 by elderly patients; ICC of 0.89 to 0.90 by elderly healthy subjects).

## Validity

A high correlation between the Box and Block Test and the Minnesota Rate of Manipulation Test - Subtest Placing has been confirmed by Cromwell (1976) with a result of r=0.91.

Further correlational analysis was performed with an independence measurement (SMAF; Functional Autonomy Measurement System; Hébert et al., 1988) and with an upper limb performance test, the Action Research Arm Test (ARAT) (Desrosiers et al., 1994). The Box and Block test correlates moderately with the SMAF (r=0.42 to 0.54) and high with the ARAT (r=0.80 and 0.82).

Desrosiers et al. (1994) correlated the result of the BBT with the ordinal scores of the TEMPA, an instrument which evaluates uni- and bilateral arm function, and demonstrated moderately high correlation coefficients of r=-0.73 to r=-0.78 .

Correlation between the Nine-Hole Peg Test and Box and Block test has been shown as moderately high (-0.7) by Goodkin et al. (1988). The moderately high result suggests that both measures describe functions which may be different.

Boissy et al. (1999) compared the scores of BBT and other upper extremity function tests with hand grip strength (computed as hand ratio score) and analysed them with linear and quadratic regression. This procedure demonstrated by 15 chronic stroke patients values of r=0.87 and 0.97; $r^2$=0.75 and 0.93.

Goodkin et al. (1988) demonstrated sensitivity to change for the BBT with MS patients, whilst impairment scales like the Kurtzke DSS and EDDS did not indicate any progress.

Thus, in terms of construct validity, it was shown that the BBT scores correlated highly with other measures of focal disability for the arm and with the degree of impairment (grip strength), but only moderately with more global measures of disability. In addition, the BBT is sensitive to change.

## Norms

Mathiowetz et al. (1985) established norms for adults in 12 age groups ranging from 20 to 94 years. Subjects older than 60 years had less stringent inclusion criteria so that persons with some chronic health problems who could maintain a normal lifestyle were included in the study. The norms for males and females were reported separately, because they found two age groups (45-49 years; 60-64 years) where the otherwise relatively small difference between both sexes were significant.

Desrosiers et al. (1994) conducted a study with 360 subjects to establish norms for persons above an age of 60 years.

Norms are also available for children (Smith, 1961).

### 3.2.6. Purpose

Mathiowetz et al. (1985) recommended the BBT for evaluation of adult individuals with deficits in manual dexterity. In addition, the availability of normative data allow a comparison of patient's results with norms.

Goodkin et al. (1988), emphasised the advantages of the Box and Block test: standardised, reliable, rapidly administered, reproducible, sensitive to change. The tool is suitable to monitor progress of upper arm function, although the phenomenon tested is a very specific function. According to Desrosiers et al. (1994) the BBT measures unilateral gross manual dexterity.

### 3.2.7. Comments

This test is easy to construct, to learn and to apply. Its simplicity prevents problems that might occur especially when administered to young or old people and patients with additional cognitive deficits. Persons of practically any age are generally able to understand the guidelines. Testing and scoring time is rather short. Aside from its simplicity a further strength is the ratio level data provided by the test. The results can be compared with norms. Since the patient needs a certain minimum arm or hand function to transport the blocks, a floor effect can be observed with severely impaired persons.

Several authors mention the disturbing noise of the falling blocks. According to our experience, a piece of soft cushioning material, e.g. felt, on the bottom of the box reduces this drawback considerably.

The Box and Block test is frequently used in research and rehabilitation of children and adults.

# 3.3. Action Research Arm test

### 3.3.1. Idea and Theories

The Action Research Arm Test (ARAT), developed by Lyle (1981), is based on the Upper Extremity Function Test (U.E.F.T., Carroll, 1965). The U.E.F.T. had been developed to monitor upper extremity function, related to every-day-activities. The test was also intended to have predictive validity, which had been demonstrated as insufficient for muscle tests and range of motion assessments among chronic patients. The idea underlying the test construction was, that complex upper extremity movements could be reduced to certain patterns, i.e. grasp, pinch, grip of the hand etc. The instrument was intended to be simple, quick and suitable for outpatients. Each of the 33 items of the original U.E.F.T. was rated according to an ordinal 4-point scale.

Lyle intended to shorten the test, but tried to stay close to Carroll´s guidelines. In addition to some small alterations due to simplification or availability of testing material, he changed some major characteristics of the U.E.F.T.

The main changes were:

- number of items were reduced to 19
- items were ordered in four subtests which were thought to represent the main aspects of upper limb function: Grasp, Grip, Pinch, Gross movement
- each subtest was structured hierarchically (Guttmann scaled) to save testing time
- all objects can be placed appropriately for the side being tested instead of standardised starting and target positions, although the distance between start and end of the movement should be as stated in the task description

The Guttman scaled shortened version of the U.E.F.T. was named Action Research Arm Test. The information presented in this chapter relates to the ARAT.

### 3.3.2. Description

All items have to be performed unilaterally with the patient in a seated position. Equipment consists of two platforms, the lower one on table level and the upper shelf appr. 30 cm high. Different objects such as wooden cubes, metal tubes, marble, ball bearing etc. are also necessary (see table 1 and 2).

Subtest „grasp" covers grasping objects of different shape and weight and raising them to the higher shelf.

Subtest „grip" contains the tasks of pouring water from one tumbler to another involving pronation, transferring vertically positioned tubes further away and placing a metal washer over a peg.

Subtest „pinch" offers the patient a marble and a ball-bearing which have first to be picked up and then to be placed on top of the shelf with various finger combinations.

Subtest „gross movement" requires movements without objects: the patient is asked to reach the back of the head, the top of the head and the mouth with his/her hand.

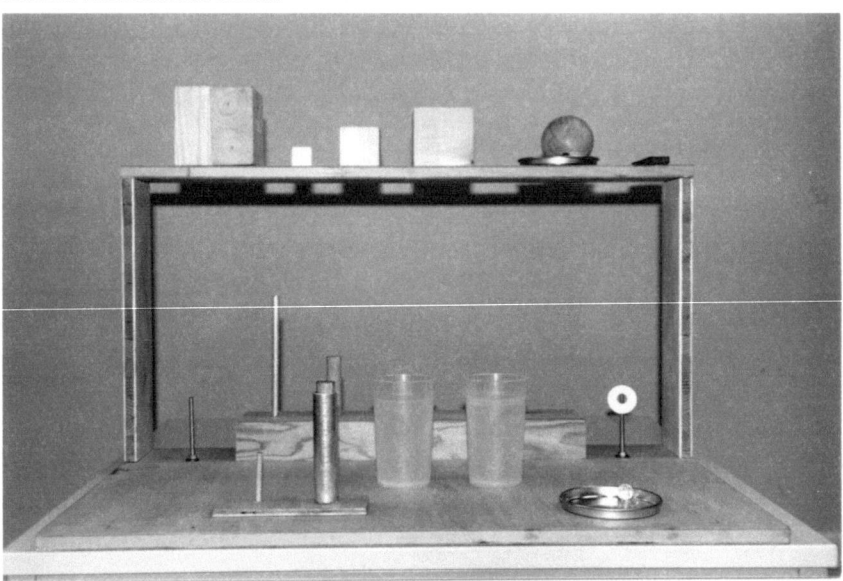

Figure: Action Research Arm test - Material

## Size of the test construction of the
## Action Research Arm test (ARAT)

| test material | Size | item |
|---|---|---|
| lower platform | 72 cm x 44 cm x 1.6 cm | |
| distance to the ground | table height of 75 cm plus 1.6 cm (= height of the wooden platform) | |
| upper shelf | 72 cm x 10 cm, distance to the lower platform 37.6 cm | |
| height of chair | 46 cm | |
| plank for the target points of the tubes | 5.0 cm x 10.0 cm x 44.0 cm | Grip 2, 3 |
| wooden peg for the large tube (starting position) | round wooden pole 2.0 cm diameter, height 13.3 cm (fixed on a mobile basis/platform) | Grip 2 |
| bolt without head, for the small iron tube (starting position) | round wooden pole 0.6 cm diameter, height 5.8 cm (fixed on a mobile basis/platform) | Grip 3 |
| bolt in plank (target position) | round wooden pole 2.0 cm, height 7.8 cm | Grip 2 |
| bolt in plank (target position) | round wooden pole 0.6 cm, height 6.2 cm | Grip 3 |
| tobacco tin lid | diameter 10 cm, rim of 1 cm | Grasp 5, Grip 4, Pinch 1-6 |
| finishing nail (or wooden peg; target position for the washer) | height 8.3 cm, diameter 0.6 cm | Grip 4 |

### Objects of the
### Action Research Arm test (ARAT)

| object | size | item |
|---|---|---|
| wooden block | 10.0 cm x 10.0 cm x 10.0 cm | Grasp 1 |
| wooden block | 7.5 cm x 7.5 cm x 7.5 cm | Grasp 4 |
| wooden block | 5.0 cm x 5.0 cm x 5.0 cm | Grasp 3 |
| wooden block | 2.5 cm x 2.5 cm x 2.5 cm | Grasp 2 |
| large metal pipe/tube (aluminium) | diameter 2.5 cm; length 11.3 cm | Grip 2 |
| small metal pipe/tube (aluminium) | diameter 1.0 cm; length 16.0 cm | Grip 3 |
| wooden ball | diameter 7.0 cm | Grasp 5 |
| marble | diameter 1.5 cm | Pinch 2, 5, 6 |
| stone | 10.8 x 2.5 x 1 cm | Grasp 6 |
| ball bearing | 6 mm diameter | Pinch 1, 3, 4 |
| 2 plastic tumbler | 12 x 7 cm diameter | Grip 1 |
| washer | outer diameter 3.5 cm, inner diameter 1.2 cm | Grip 4 |

### 3.3.3. Performance

Each extremity is assessed separately. The assessor demonstrates the tasks until the patient is aware of what he/she is expected to do. It is recommended that the patient starts with the less or non-impaired limb. The patient always starts with the first item of each subtest and continues according to the scoring guidelines. Any of the objects are to be placed appropriately for the side being tested, the objects are presented one by one.

### 3.3.4. Scoring

An ordinal 4-point scale is applied to each item, the maximum score for each extremity is 57 points. A score of „0" is given if the patient is not able to perform any part of the task; for a score of „1" he/she should be able to lift the object completely from the platform. A score of „2" describes a function which is performed fully, but clumsily or with great difficulty. A score of „3" is allocated when the item is performed normally. The score is not based on a comparison between the extremities. The hierarchical structure of the subtests implies that a full score in the first item predicts success in the following items (i.e. the easier ones) of the same subtest. Therefore, a patient who solves the first item perfectly will gain the full score for the complete subtest without having to perform them. A patient who receives a score of „0" for the first and most difficult item, will be presented with the easiest item next. If he/she fails here, a score of „0" is allocated for this subtest. If the second item can be performed at least partially (score $\geq$ 1), the patient continues with the following items as indicated for that subtest. Any patient who scores either 1 or 2 on the first item, has to perform all items of that subtest.

### 3.3.5. Test properties
Each subtest internally fulfils the statistical criteria of a coefficient of reproducibility of at least 0.9 and a coefficient of scalability of well above 0.6.

### Reliability
Several studies revealed a very high interrater-reliability with values over 0.95 (Lyle, 1981; Carroll, 1965; Hsieh et al., 1998, ICC). Test-retest reliability and interrater reliability is very high (0.98 and 0.99) according to the findings of Lyle, 1981 (cited by De Weerdt & Harrison, 1985).

### Validity
The ARAT is well studied in terms of construct validity and is characterised by high correlation coefficients of its scores with scores of the arm sections of the Motricity Index (r=0.87; Hsieh et al., 1998), the Motor Assessment Scale (r=0.96; Hsieh et al., 1998), and with the Fugl-Meyer Test (rho=0.91 and 0.94; De Weerdt & Harrison, 1985). Since the ARAT correlates well with validated impairment measures, Hsieh et al. (1998) suggested, that the ARAT scores may also indicate upper extremity motor impairment.

The test also correlates with functional ADL-Scales (0.55 to 0.60). Desrosiers et al. (1994) revealed a moderate correlation with the SMAF, which represents an independence measure (r=0.32 to 0.48). Criterion validity in terms of arm activity limitations has been demonstrated in correlational analysis using the Box and Block Test (r=0.80 and 0.82; Desrosiers et al., 1994) and the TEMPA (ordinal scores r=-0.90 to -0.95; Desrosiers et al., 1994b). In addition, the ARAT scores were moderately correlated with Motor Activity Log (MAL) scores that reflect the use of the paretic arm and hand during activities of daily living among chronic stroke patients as assessed by a semistructured interview (Spearman rho=0.63; van der Lee et al., 2004). Sensitivity to change has been shown by De Weerdt & Harrison (1985) and Hsueh & Hsieh (2002).

### 3.3.6. Purpose

The ARAT is able to assess the level of upper limb function following cortical damage. In addition, it can be applied to monitor progress, e.g. as related to treatment in a clinical or research context. Additionally, Lyle suggested that patients may be classified in prognostic groups based on ARAT results (De Weerdt & Harrison, 1885).

### 3.3.7. Comments

The ARAT assesses limitations of upper limb function quickly and easily. The tasks afford the manipulation of objects, but do not reflect activities of daily living, although the ordinal score correlates with functional ADL-scales.

One major drawback of the assessment is that the testing material has to be purpose-built.

# 4. Test properties of the manual-based use of the arm assessment scales

## 4.1. Reliability and validity study

In general, users of the arm assessment scales rely on original publications for reference, which focus on psychometric properties rather than provide the necessary detailed guidance for performance and scoring of the test. Manuals specifically addressing issues of performance and scoring of motor scales could facilitate a standardised test application and thereby communication and comparison of research results across clinical centres. Based on original publications, the authors prepared detailed manuals for both performance (test administration) and scoring of three arm function tests. The reliability and validity study (Platz et al., 2005) set out to investigate whether reliable assessment of arm function with these tests could be achieved between different clinical centres and the extent to which the constructs addressed by the arm function tests were congruent with other neurological tests of impairment and activity limitation. Patients with upper limb paresis resulting from either stroke, multiple sclerosis, or traumatic brain injury were included.

Fifty-six patients entered the study, of which 37 had had a stroke. Thirty-three of these patients had had an ischaemic stroke, 3 an intracerebral, and 1 a subarachnoidal haemorrhage.

Regarding the order of the arm motor tests, the following sequence was used for all patients: the Fugl-Meyer test, arm section (FM) was followed by the Action Research Arm test (ARAT), which was followed by the Box and Block test (BBT). Within each of the tests, each item was performed firstly with the non- or less affected arm to ensure sufficient comprehension of the tasks and then with the (more) affected arm. The performance of all tests was videotaped to ensure undivided attention could be paid to the scoring process. Using a large mirror both frontal and sagittal planes were simultaneously videotaped. The performance of the (more) affected arm only was scored, based on video information.

Data sets from 12 patients were used for training, i.e. open discussion regarding test administration and scoring among the project partners. For the data collection proper, data sets from 44 patients were scored as follows: on first assessment, two raters scored the performance of each patient independently from each other and blinded to each others scores: one rater from the clinical centre who collected the data, and the other as the "central rater". These data sets were used for the inter-rater reliability analysis. Test-retest reliability was studied over a period of 7 days. The data sets from 23 of the 44 patients mentioned above, who were available for assessment on a second occasion after 7 days, were used for the analysis of test-retest reliability. These data sets were scored by the rater from each clinical centre who collected the data. Raters were blinded to the data collected at first assessment.

## 4.2. Reliability

The reliability data demonstrated that high to very high inter-rater and test-retest reliability could be achieved with the manual, described in chapter 5, for all total and subtest scores of the three motor tests (ICC for interrater reliability $> 0.96$; for test-retest reliability: $ICC_{total\ motor\ scores} > 0.96$, $ICC_{motor\ subtest\ scores} > 0.89$). Previously, equally high reliability had been demonstrated when these test were evaluated in single centre studies. In the current project, assessment of sensation, passive joint motion, or joint pain was equally reliable across facilities (ICC $> 0.96$) and thus improved as compared to a previous report (ICC ranging from 0.61 to 0.85 (Sanford et al., 1993)). Over time, however, assessment of sensation was somewhat less reliable (ICC $= 0.81$).

It is important to note that the degree of reproducibility reported in the literature within single centres, could now also be achieved across facilities from three different European countries. The manual developed can thus promote the comparability of arm motor assessment across centres and can be used for single and follow-up assessments of individuals with arm paresis due to lesions of the upper motor neuron. The manual could thus be introduced to further standardise established outcome measures in clinical quality management programs across centres and be used in multicenter clinical trials.

It is highlighted that both provision of the detailed test manual and training of data collection centres were necessary to achieve the required degree of standardisation across facilities. In addition, due to the separation of test administration and video-based scoring, the assessors could give undivided attention to both processes.

For routine clinical purposes, it is also important to note that reproducibility of results was independent of the condition that caused the arm paresis. Reliability coefficients were almost identical for patients with stroke, multiple sclerosis, or traumatic brain injury.

## 4.3. Validity

It was of further interest to explore the association between the constructs measured by these arm motor tests. Further insight to construct validity, as provided by correlational analyses, might assist in the selection of tests for specific purposes. The high correlation between the FM (arm motor section), ARAT and BBT (0.900 -0.935) suggests that the association between the constructs they assess is considerable. Similarly high correlations have previously been documented for the FM and ARAT ($r_s$ = 0.91 to 0.94 (De Weerdt and Harrison, 1985)). While it can be argued that the three arm motor tests assess a similar construct, e.g. 'arm function', it is nevertheless conceivable that specific information may be obtained from these tests, especially at item or subtest level. It appears that the FM primarily assesses impairment in terms of loss or abnormality of movement, i.e. the inability to perform movements in accordance with specified joint motion pattern, whilst both the ARAT and BBT assess primarily activity limitations, i.e. a patient's functional loss when interacting with the environment by means of the upper limb. Further research is warranted to elucidate the potentially different information content of the Fugl-Meyer test and Action Research Arm test at the level of individual items and subtests.

In terms of resolution, the FM could - in contrast to the other two arm motor tests - detect differences throughout the spectrum of motor dysfunction of the study population. Compared to the ARAT and BBT, the FM was least affected by floor or ceiling effects, while the ARAT showed

both some floor and ceiling effects, i.e. it did not differentiate well
between subjects at either the lower or upper end of the spectrum. The
BBT had a considerable floor effect, hence it was not able to differentiate
among subjects with severe impairment (i.e. FM (arm motor section) score
< 19).

In terms of practicality, the FM can be performed almost without test
material, while the ARAT has to be purpose-built. The latter has, however,
the great advantage to be hierarchically organized, which reduces
administration and scoring time. The test material of the BBT also has to
be purpose-built. The advantage of this test is that it takes only a few
minutes to administer.

The study further addressed the question whether the arm motor tests
provided additional or redundant information compared with other tests of
impairment and activity limitations.

Resistance to passive movement, as assessed with the Ashworth Scale,
showed only a moderate correlation with motor function when assessed
with any of the three arm motor tests ($r < 0.45$), suggesting that scores on
the Ashworth were not closely related to active motor function. This is
perhaps not surprising, given the fact that the Ashworth Scale merely
indicated resistance to passive movement (at the elbow joint). The data
thus supported the use of arm motor function tests in addition to the
Ashworth Scale.

A relatively crude measure of paresis (Motricity Index) and a more global
measure of neurological impairment (Hemispheric Stroke Scale) showed a
high to moderately high correlation with the arm motor tests ($r = 0.735$ to
$0.861$ and $0.631$ to $0.714$ respectively). This indicates that arm motor
function, as assessed with the three arm motor tests, is strongly related to
paresis and somewhat less to overall severity of neurological impairment.
Thus, the separate assessment of arm function, in addition to these more
general impairments, might be warranted.

Surprisingly, the correlation between arm motor function and patients'
ability to cope with usual activities of daily living as assessed on the
Barthel Idex was very low if not absent ($r = 0.095$ to $0.152$). In an earlier
smaller study with 18 stroke patients, a moderate correlation between the
Barthel Index and the FM (arm section) had been documented ($r_s = 0.60$,
Filiatrault et al., 1991). The inconsistent and low correlation might

indicate that arm dysfunction does not necessarily imply dependence on caregivers for basic activities of daily living (ADL). Patients might - quite independently of severity of arm dysfunction - learn to cope with ADL, e.g. by acquiring compensatory strategies and using technical aids. Since all patients of the study population were recruited from neurorehabilitation referral centres, the data might reflect a situation where patients have already been involved in this adaptation process. However, it is important to note that the Modified Barthel Index does not address the costs of such adaptation (e.g. a change of wardrobe to match reduced dressing skills), nor does it address issues such as pain or fatigue associated with ADL. Thus, since the Modified Barthel Index addresses a patient's ability to cope with ADL (which may involve compensatory strategies), the information derived from it may mask true needs for treatment, recovery or effects of treatment, which are essential to be monitored. To this purpose, specific upper limb outcome measures are required.

## 4.4. Summary

For many clinical motor scales a detailed user manual is not available. Such a manual was developed for the Fugl-Meyer test (arm section), the Action Research Arm test, and the Box and Block test. The manual- and video-based assessment of stroke, multiple sclerosis, and traumatic brain injury patients enabled standardisation and thus assured reliable and valid arm motor assessment across facilities and over time (i.e. with retesting). All three tests are suitable for both single and repeated assessments of individuals with arm paresis due to an upper motor neuron lesion. The total motor scores of these tests provide similar information that is closely related to the degree of paresis. The Fugl-Meyer test (arm section) was least affected by floor or ceiling effects. The three arm motor tests provide information that is (1) not identical to information provided by a more generic scales of neurological impairment and (2) quite independent of a person's ability to cope with basic activities of daily living.

# 5. Manual for the use of the arm assessment scales

## 5.1. General testing recommendations

The following general testing recommendations mostly refer to all three tests.

### 5.1.1. Starting position
The patient is seated on a normal chair without arm rests. Except in one item of the Fugl-Meyer test („Hand to lumbar spine"), the patient is asked to sit with the back against the backrest to avoid compensatory spinal extension.

In patients who are seated in a wheelchair and who have difficulty transferring themselves, the patient is allowed to remain in her/his wheelchair. Sitting on a treatment table/plinth may also be appropriate.

Patients need to start from the correct position, but if this causes pain / discomfort, the position is approximated as far as comfortable and a note is made of the adaptation required.

### 5.1.2. General performance guidelines
Video recording is advised to clarify details between assessors and to support the scoring process which has not necessary to be simultaneous to the testing performance. The zoom function of the camera is recommended when evaluating the distal parts of the arm.

Work with a minimum of upper body clothing.

Use a mirror to provide the assessor with a second plane of view. The size of the mirror should be sufficient to show the important body parts (i.e. arm flexed in the shoulder joint and extended in the elbow joint) without adapting the position of the mirror during each task. We recommend a mirror of appr. 70 cm width and 150 cm height positioned on the affected side in an angle of 45° to 70° depending both on the body part which has to be captured and on the width of the mirror. A second camera may also be used to obtain a second plane.

The scores are based on sensomotor abilities *per se*. Therefore, ensure that the patient is rested and that the instructions are well-understood.

Start each task with the non- or less affected side.

Do not ask the patient to perform any item with both sides simultaneously.

### 5.1.3. Instructions to the patient

Take care to ensure that the patient fully understands the instructions. The strategy employed depends on the patient's abilities.

Firstly, the assessor explains the movement, using demonstration and verbal instruction. The patient then copies the movement with the non- or less affected side. If required, the assessor guides the patient, using passive or active-assisted movement.

Secondly, the assessor demonstrates the movement for the affected side (we may not assume that the patient is able to mirror the movement without further instruction). Instruction and/or guided movement are provided as needed. Corrections are offered if and when required.

It is also important that the patient is given the opportunity to demonstrate the best possible performance. Sufficient opportunity for repetition should be allowed, but care should be taken that the patient does not become fatigued or trained.

### 5.1.4. General scoring guidelines

The tests examine both left and right side for all sections. Both sides may be recorded using video. Scoring will cover the affected side only by the Fugl-Meyer Test, both sides by the Box and Block Test and the Action Research Arm Test.

The analysis of the movement patterns alone and not muscle activation is the basis for the scores, since the latter cannot be validly assessed without additional EMG equipment.

# 5.2. Manual for the Fugl-Meyer test, arm section

## 5.2.1. General remarks

### Equipment

The following testing objects have to be organised:

- reflex hammer
- paper sheet, folded ¼ A4 (A6)
- pencil
- cylinder shaped object/can, diameter 3.0 cm, i.e. bottle of tip-ex fluid
- tennis ball

### Instructions to the patient

*Original text*

As in all other performance tests using this method, the patient must be meticulously instructed and it may often be an advantage to use mime as well as verbal means of instruction in order to minimise perceptual difficulties. It may often facilitate the evaluation procedure if the patient initially performs the required manoeuvre with the non-affected arm.

*Comments*

Ensure that the patient does not deviate from the instructions and take care that the patient only receives assistance to reach the starting position or to perform the movement in cases when the score does not refer to these details. When the examiner supports the patient to get into the starting position, a few seconds may be required to allow the limb to return to its resting position before proceeding to active movements (otherwise the latter could be mistaken for a synergy). In some items the score is based on the ability of the patient to maintain this resting position in a joint during the movement performed in other joints.

### Starting position

Some scores are dependent on the patient's ability to reach and/or maintain the starting position independently. Do not assist the patient in these items of the Fugl-Meyer test (FM).

In other items, the assessor is allowed to support the patient to reach the starting position. In these cases, assist the patient to get into the starting position and ask him/her to start the movement after a period of appr. 3 seconds. During this short period, the assessor observes, whether the patient is able to maintain the position or not. However, if the patient loses the required starting position before the movement begins but there is no change during the movement (joint position at the start of movement = joint position at the end of movement), he/she will not be penalised (apply this guideline to: shoulder flexion 0-90°, abduction 0-90°).

## Recording passive range of motion (RoM)

Although the FM includes the assessment of the passive range of motion as section „J", it is recommended to start with this particular section. Nevertheless, it may be helpful to repeat the evaluation of relevant passive RoM. The passive RoM (section „J") is recorded on video for both left and right side to enable the assessor to determine whether active RoM covers the full passive RoM and hence to differentiate between a score of 1 or 2 for items related to activity. If active RoM covers passive RoM (even when passive RoM is limited), a score of 2 will be allocated.

For definition of joint motion, the standards of the American Academy of Orthopaedic Surgeons (1965) are used.

## Each task separately

Do not connect any of the Fugl-Meyer motor part tasks, except the "finger flexion" and "finger extension" - each task should be performed as a distinctive unit. Ensure there is a clear interval (e.g. 3 seconds) between one test and the next.

## Scoring specifics

If the patient performs the task more than once, the score should be given for the best performance.

The score refers not to the ability of the patient to repeat a movement several times, except when it is mentioned explicitly in the description of the scoring procedure.

Some items of the Fugl-Meyer Test are scored with regard to the passive range of motion. In these cases the examiner is asked to repeat the assessment of passive range of motion when assessing the motor item. The score is then based on this comparison.

Some scores of the Fugl-Meyer Test are allocated by comparing performance of the affected side to the non-affected side. However, in cases where the other side is less or more severely impaired (as often seen by MS and TBI patients), this procedure does not yield a meaningful description of motor function of the extremity concerned. Instead, in patients who present with two affected upper limbs, motor performance should be scored by comparing the primarily assessed extremity with regular non-affected motor performance.

## 5.2.2. How to perform and score the Fugl-Meyer test - specific remarks

Remarks are divided as follows:
1.  derived from the <u>original text </u>(item per item)
2.  <u>comments</u> that further clarify what has been implicated by the original text, and
3.  <u>added specifications</u> for any test item where it was felt that the original text did not specify all aspects necessary to collect data in a standardised way.

Additionally, statements and recommendations concerning special scoring techniques are included for those assessors using video. These remarks are not mentioned in general, but with regard to each item. For those who perform and score simultaneously, this information is not relevant.

# Fugl-Meyer Arm score

## A.      Shoulder/ Elbow/ Forearm

## I      Reflex activity

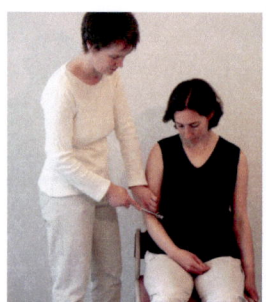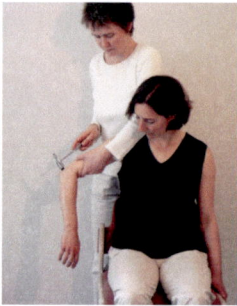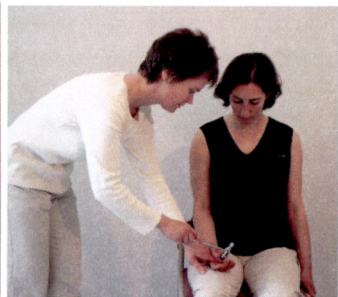

| **A. Shoulder-Elbow-Forearm** (patient sitting) | |
|---|---|
| **I REFLEX-ACTIVITY** *Biceps, Triceps, Fingerflexors* | - no reflex-activity ☐ 0 <br> - reflex-activity in biceps <br>   and/or fingerflexors ☐ 2 <br><br> - no reflex-activity ☐ 0 <br> - reflex-activity in extensors ☐ 2 |

## Performance

*Original text*

The biceps-, triceps-, and finger-flexor reflexes are elicited.

*Added specifications*

Show repeatability of each reflex.

- for m. biceps brachii, the patient's hand is lying on his/her lap, forearm in supination.
- for mm. flexor digitorum, the patient's hand is lying on his/her lap, forearm in supination. The assessor places the index finger on the volar side of the proximal phalanges and taps own finger with reflex hammer.
- for m. triceps brachii, the upper arm is abducted by the assessor, allowing the elbow to fall into passive flexion.

## Scoring

*Original text*

0: no reflex activity
2: reflex activity can be elicited in flexor and/or the extensor.

*Comments*

Note that for "flexors" either the biceps or the finger flexor reflex is sufficient.

**II      Volitional movement can be performed within the dynamic flexor and/or extensor synergies**

**a      Flexor Synergy**

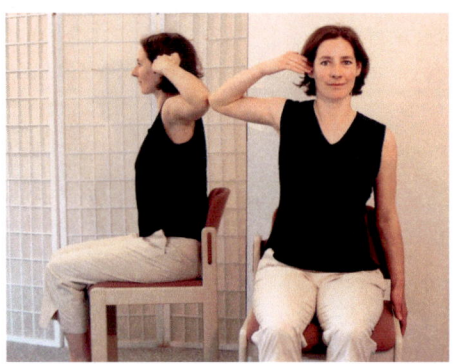

| A. Shoulder-Elbow-Forearm | | | |
|---|---|---|---|
| **II VOLITIONAL MOVEMENTS WITHIN DYNAMIC SYNERGIES** (patient sitting with the back against the backrest) *a) Flexor synergy*: "hand to your (ipsilateral) ear" with shoulder retraction | | | |

|  |  | none | partial | perfect |
|---|---|---|---|---|
| forearm | supination: | ☐ 0 | ☐ 1 | ☐ 2 |
| elbow | flexion: | ☐ 0 | ☐ 1 | ☐ 2 |
|  | outw rotation: | ☐ 0 | ☐ 1 | ☐ 2 |
| shoulder | abduction (90°) | ☐ 0 | ☐ 1 | ☐ 2 |
|  | elevation: | ☐ 0 | ☐ 1 | ☐ 2 |
|  | retraction: | ☐ 0 | ☐ 1 | ☐ 2 |

## *Performance*

*Original text*

The seated patient is instructed by voluntary action of muscles of the affected arm to bring his forearm fully supinated to the ear of the affected side, the elbow fully flexed, the shoulder abducted to at least 90° outwards rotated, retracted and elevated.

*Comments*

It is important that all components are realised at the end of the movement. The fingers are in a natural, i.e. somewhat flexed, position, the movement is performed utilising the maximum range of motion (RoM) in the elbow and shoulder joints.

## *Scoring*

*Original text*

0: the specific detail (see score sheet) cannot be performed at all
1: the detail can be performed only partly
2: the detail is performed faultlessly

*Comments*

Note that spinal lateral flexion may compensate for shoulder abducttion.

The components of both synergies (i.e. a and b) are evaluated at the end of the movement. Do not score separate abilities during the trajectory of the movement.

**b      Extensor Synergy**

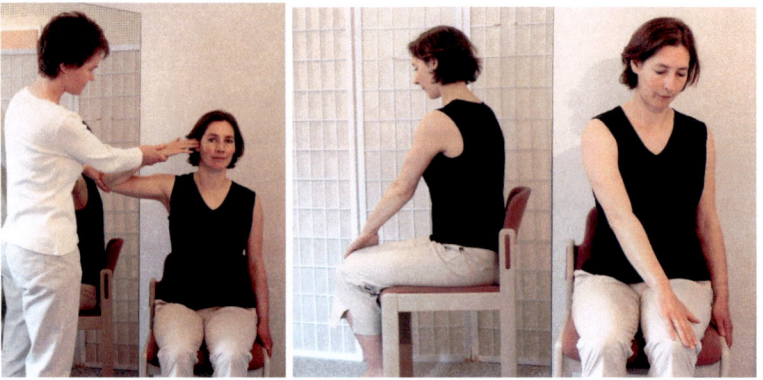

| b) *Extensor synergy:* "knuckles on contralateral knee" from <u>flexor synergy</u> (with support, if needed) Make sure that the knees are placed apart. | | | | |
|---|---|---|---|---|
| forearm | pronation: | ☐ 0 | ☐ 1 | ☐ 2 |
| elbow | extension: | ☐ 0 | ☐ 1 | ☐ 2 |
| shoulder | adduction + int rotation: | ☐ 0 | ☐ 1 | ☐ 2 |

## *Performance*

*Original text*

The seated patient is instructed to adduct/internally rotate the shoulder, extend his arm towards the unaffected knee, forearm pronated. The starting position should be that of full flexor synergy. If the patient cannot actively attain this position, the arm may be passively „placed" therein. Care should be taken to avoid letting the patient substitute gravitational help for muscle activity. Some patients, eager to cooperate, may for instance rotate the thorax or pendulate the affected arm. To assess if the motion is actively performed by the patient, it may now and then be necessary to palpate the pectoralis major and/or the triceps brachii tendons.

*Added specifications*

The knees of the patient should have some space between them to require full extension and adduction. The patient is asked to put the palmar surface of the hand (not the thumb) on the contralateral knee.

The focus of this test is *active movement* - palpation is omitted.

If necessary, support the patient to reach the starting position including all components and then ensure that the patient's arm is not "dropped".

## *Scoring*

*Original text*

The criteria for scoring are identical to those listed above.

*Comments*

The ability to pronate is judged with regard to the reached end position on the knee and not with regard to complete RoM.

The components of both synergies (i.e. a and b) are evaluated at the end of the movement. Do not score separated abilities during the trajectory of the movement.

**III     Volitional motion performed mixing dynamic flexor and extensor synergy**

**a     Hand to lumbar spine**

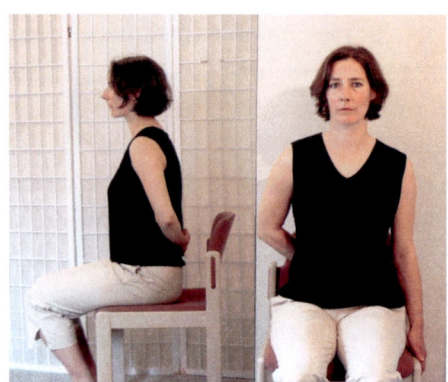

| A. Shoulder-Elbow-Forearm | |
|---|---|
| **III VOLITIONAL MOVEMENTS WITHIN A MIX OF DYNAMIC SYNERGIES**<br><br>*a) Hand to lumbar spine*<br>"bring your hand on your back"<br>Patient seated towards the front of the chair. | - hand not behind<br>  spina iliaca ant. sup.          □ 0<br>- hand behind spina iliaca ant. sup.,<br>  without any gravitational trick   □ 1<br>- perfect                             □ 2 |

## Performance

*Original text*

Actively position the affected hand on the lumbar spine.

*Added specifications*

The patient has to be seated towards the front of the chair before performing the task. Ensure patient maintains an upright position to avoid compensatory movements. The examiner is allowed to give some manual guidance to facilitate the upright position. The hand reaches the back with its dorsal side.

## Scoring

*Original text*

0: the specific detail cannot be performed at all
1: the hand should, without any gravitational tricks, pass the anterior-superior iliac spine
2: the detail is performed faultlessly

*Comments*

A score of 0 is allocated, if the patient does not get past the anterior-superior iliac spine or if he/she overcomes it only by compensatory movements.

**b      Shoulder flexion 0 to 90°**

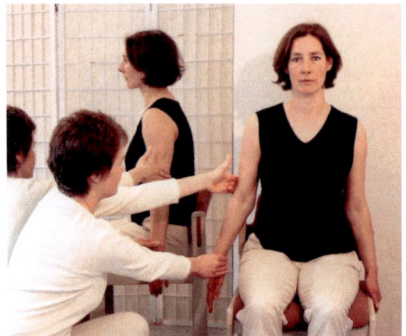 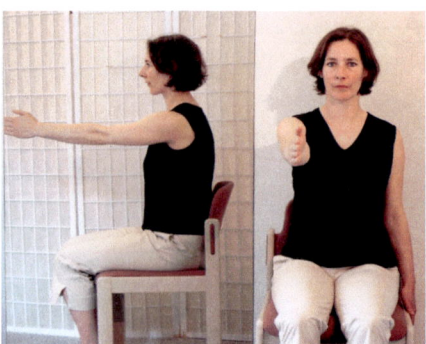

| | |
|---|---|
| *b) Shoulder flexion 0° to 90°*<br>elbow extended, forearm in mid-position<br>"Bring your extended arm up, thumb upwards".<br>The examiner may assist the patient to get into the starting position. | - arm immediately in abduction<br>   or elbow in flexion   ☐ 0<br>- arm not immediately in<br>   abduction and/or elbow<br>   in flexion   ☐ 1<br>- perfect   ☐ 2 |

## *Performance*

| *Original text* | *Added specifications* |
|---|---|
| Flex the shoulder to 90° in a pure flexion motion. The elbow must be fully extended throughout the total required range of motion, the forearm in the midposition between pro- and supination. | The examiner may assist the seated patient to get into the starting position (shoulder 0° in all degrees of freedom, elbow fully extended, forearm in midposition, arm hanging to the side of the patient / chair). |

## *Scoring*

*Original text*

0: If, at the start of the motion, the arm is immediately abducted or the elbow flexed.

1: If, in later phases of the motion, shoulder abduction and/or elbow flexion occurs.

*Added specification*

A score of 1 is allocated if the patient cannot cover the full passive RoM.

**c      Pronation-supination of the forearm, the elbow flexed to 90°**

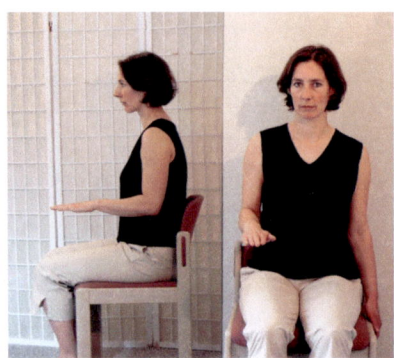 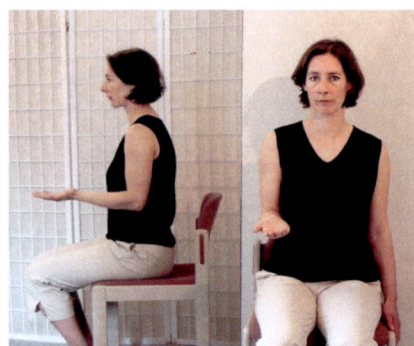

| *c) Pro-Supination of the forearm* | |
|---|---|
| elbow flexed 90°, shoulder 0° | - starting position impossible |
| The patient has to reach this posi-tion without support. Score against passive RoM. | and/or no pro-supination    ☐ 0 |
| | - starting position possible and kept during the move- |
| Beware of any compensation in the glenohumeral joint. | ment, limited pro-supi-nation    ☐ 1 |
| | - perfect    ☐ 2 |

## Performance

*Original text*

Pronation-supination of the forearm, the elbow joint actively flexed to about 90°, the shoulder joint at 0° (all degrees of freedom).

*Comments*

Ensure that shoulder and elbow joints are kept in the starting position, i.e. elbow close to the trunk.

## Scoring

*Original text*

0: If the correct position of the shoulder and the elbow can not be obtained by the patient and/or pro-supination can not be performed at all.

1: If active pro-supination can be performed even within a very limited range of motion and at the same time the shoulder and the elbow joints are correctly positioned.

*Comments*

Repeat the evaluation of passive RoM in this (indicated) position in order to decide whether the patient is able to cover the complete passive RoM or not.

**IV      Volitional movements are performed with little or no synergy dependence**

**a      Shoulder abduction 0 to 90°**

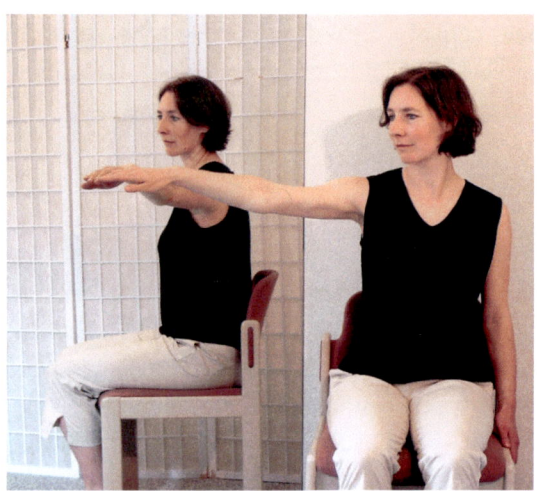

| A. Shoulder-Elbow-Forearm | |
|---|---|
| **IV VOLITIONAL MOVEMENTS WITH LITTLE OR NO SYNERGY DEPENDENCE**<br><br>*a) Shoulder abduction 0 - 90°*<br>elbow fully extended and forearm pronated<br>The examiner may assist the patient to get into the starting position. | - arm immediately supinated and/or elbow flexed ☐ 0<br>- motion only partly or elbow is flexed or the forearm can not be kept in the pronated position ☐ 1<br>- perfect ☐ 2 |

### Performance

*Original text*

The seated patient is instructed to abduct the shoulder to 90° in a pure abduction motion. The elbow fully extended (0°) and the forearm pronated.

*Comments*

Palm of hand faces down.

*Added specifications*

The examiner may assist the patient to get into the starting position if needed.

### Scoring

*Original text*

1: If the motion can be performed only partly or if, during the motion, the elbow is flexed or the forearm can not be kept in the pronated position.
2: No initial flexion of the elbow should be tolerated nor should any deviation from the pronated forearm position be allowed.

*Added specifications*

Initial flexion of the elbow or any initial deviation of the pronated forearm is scored with 0.

**b      Shoulder flexion 90 to 180°**

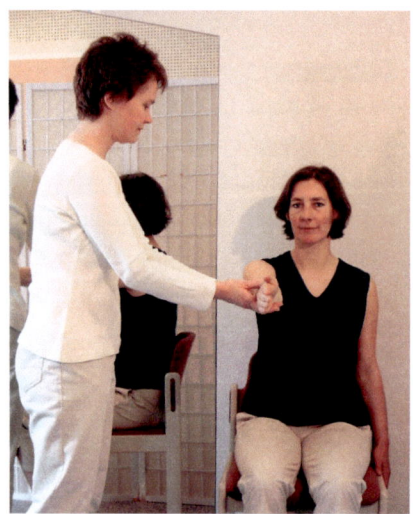 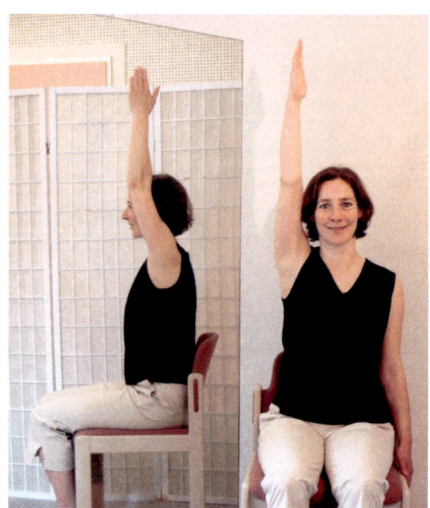

| | |
|---|---|
| *b) Shoulder flexion 90° to 180°*<br>arm in 0° abduction, elbow extended and forearm in midposition<br>"Bring extended arm up, thumb up"<br>The examiner may assist the patient to get into the starting position. | - arm immediately in abd. or<br>  elbow flexed                                              ☐ 0<br>- arm not immediately in<br>  abduction and/or elbow<br>  in flexion                                                      ☐ 1<br>- perfect                                                          ☐ 2 |

## *Performance*

*Original text*

The seated patient is instructed to flex the shoulder in a pure flexion motion from 90° to 180°.

*Added specifications*

The examiner may assist the patient to get / place the arm in the required starting position (shoulder 90° flexion and 0° abduction). The patient is asked to move from this position.

## *Scoring*

*Original text*

0: If, at the start of the motion, the arm is immediately abducted or the elbow flexed.

1: If, in later phases of the motion, shoulder abduction and/or elbow flexion occurs.

*Added specifications*

A score of 1 is also allocated if the patient can not cover the full range of motion.

**c     Pronation-supination of the forearm, the elbow fully extended**

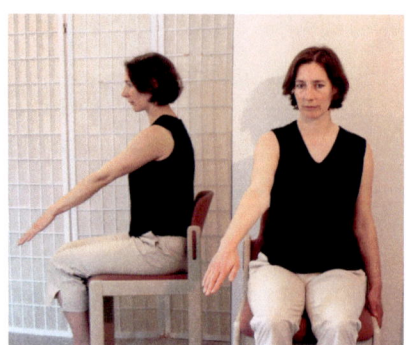 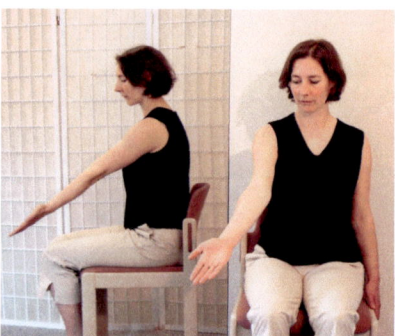

| | |
|---|---|
| <u>*c) Pro-Supination of the forearm*</u><br>shoulder 30° - 90° flexion, elbow in extension<br>The patient has to reach this position without support. Score against passive RoM.<br>Beware of any compensation in the glenohumeral joint. | - starting position impossible and/or no pro-supination   ☐ 0<br>- starting position possible and kept during the movement, limited pro-supination   ☐ 1<br>- perfect   ☐ 2 |

## *Performance*

| *Original text* | Comments |
|---|---|
| The seated patient is instructed to pro-supinate the forearm, the elbow fully extended (0°). The shoulder must be kept in a position between at least 30° and no more than 90° flexion. | The patient does not receive any physical help to come into the starting position. |

## *Scoring*

Original text

0: If the correct position of the shoulder and the elbow can not be obtained by the patient and/or pro-supination can not be performed at all.

1: If active pro-supination can be performed even within a very limited range of motion and at the same time the shoulder and the elbow joints are correctly positioned.

Comments

Care should be taken that rotation in the shoulder joint is not mistaken for pronation and supination in the radio-ulnar joints.

*Added specifications*

Repeat the evaluation of passive RoM in this indicated position in order to decide whether the patient is able to cover the complete range of motion or not.

A score of „1" (starting position kept, but limited movement) is allocated when the patient maintains the starting position for a small range of pro/supination and loses it by increasing the movement towards his/her full range of motion.

## V      Normal reflex activities

This stage, which can render the patient a maximum score of 2, is included only if the patient has a score of 6 points in stage IV.

| *A. Shoulder-Elbow-Forearm* | |
|---|---|
| **V   NORMAL REFLEX-ACTIVITIES**<br>Only assessed if in the previous section total<br>score = 6 | a) not assessed<br>   (because score of A. IV < 6) ☐ 0<br>b) assessed:<br>   - 2 of 3 reflex-activities are<br>      markedly hyperactive      ☐ 0<br>   - 1 reflex markedly hyper-<br>      active or 2 lively      ☐ 1<br>   - no hyperactive reflexes   ☐ 2 |

### Performance

*Original text*

The biceps-, triceps-, and finger-flexor reflexes are elicited.

*Added specifications*

In fact, reflex testing is done at the beginning (subtest AI) of the Fugl-Meyer Test. Scores are retained for this test item.

### Scoring

*Original text*

0: at least 2 of the 3 phasic reflexes
    are markedly hyperactive
1: one reflex markedly hyperactive
    or at least 2 reflexes lively
2: no more than one reflex lively
    and no reflexes markedly
    hyperactive

## B.     Wrist

The wrist items have to be performed with either the elbow flexed to 90° and the shoulder in 0° position or with the elbow fully extended and the shoulder slightly flexed. The examiner may assist the patient to achieve and keep these positions.

## a       Wrist stability with the elbow flexed to 90°

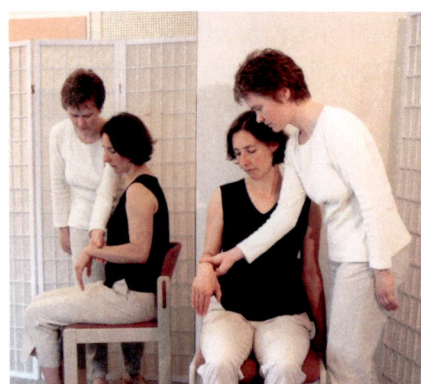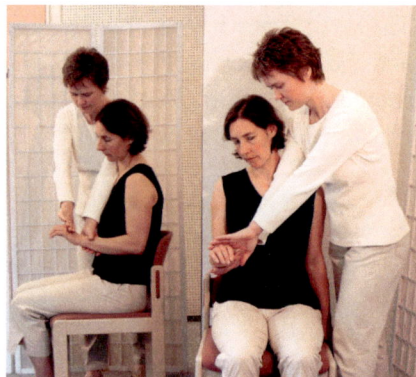

| **B. WRIST** | |
|---|---|
| *a) Wrist stability in 15° dorsal flexion*<br>shoulder 0°, elbow 90°, forearm fully pronated | - dorsiflexion to required position not possible ☐ 0<br>- required position possible, no resistance ☐ 1<br>- required position can be maintained against some (slight) resistance ☐ 2 |

## *Performance*

| *Original text* | *Comments* |
|---|---|
| Wrist stability in approximately 15° dorsal flexion is tested with the shoulder in 0° (all degrees of freedom), the elbow in 90° and the forearm fully pronated. If the elbow cannot by volitional muscle actively be brought to and kept in the required position, the examiner may assist the patient. | Apply resistance only in such cases, where the patient is able to maintain the 15° dorsiflexion against gravity. |

## *Scoring*

*Original text*

0: If the patient cannot dorsiflex the wrist in the required position.

1: If dorsifllexion can be performed but no resistance can be taken.

2: The position can be maintained against some (slight) resistance.

## b  Repeated wrist flexion and extension with the elbow flexed to 90°

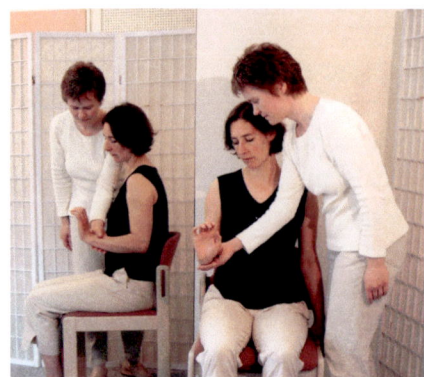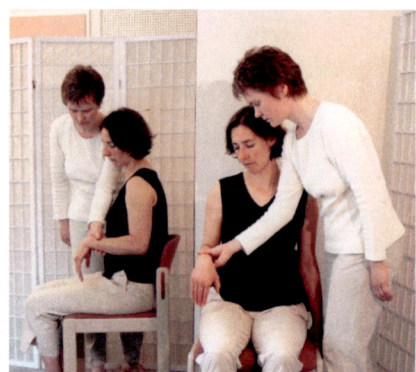

| *b) Repeated max. wrist flexion - extension* shoulder in 0°, elbow 90°, forearm pronated. Score against passive RoM. | - no active repeated movements ☐ 0<br>- active movements smaller than passive movements ☐ 1<br>- detail is fully and adequately performed ☐ 2 |
|---|---|

### Performance

*Original text*

The patient is instructed to perform repeated smooth alternating movements from maximum dorsiflexion to maximum volar flexion with the fingers somewhat flexed. The position of the shoulder-, elbow-, and radio-ulnar joints as in the foregoing manoeuvre. The examiner may support the elbow in the required position if needed.

*Comments*

During wrist extension, the fingers could be somewhat flexed.

*Added specifications*

Do not restrain the forearm. The patient is instructed to keep the forearm in the starting position.

### Scoring

*Original text*

0: Volitional movements do not occur.

1: The patient cannot actively move the wrist joint throughout the total passive range of motion.

2: Each detail is fully and adequately performed.

*Comments*

Repeat the evaluation of passive range of motion in this indicated position in order to decide whether the patient is able to cover the complete passive range of motion or not. If active RoM covers passive RoM (even when passive RoM is limited), a score of 2 will be allocated.

To allocate a score of „1", the movements have to be repeated in both directions.

Do not confuse release of spasticity for a flicker of active movement.

**c      Wrist stability with the elbow fully extended**

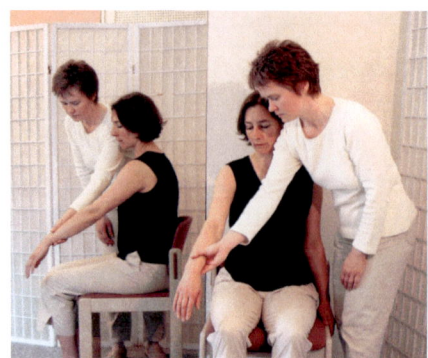
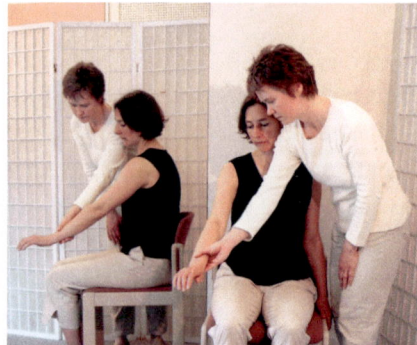

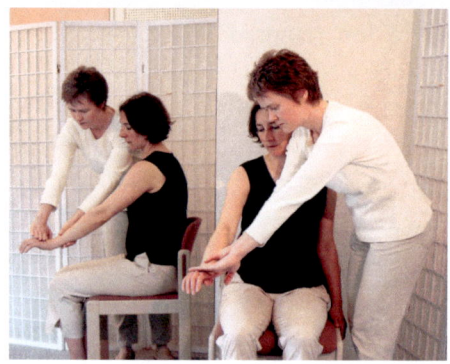

| *c) Wrist stability in 15° dorsiflexion* shoulder slightly flexed and/or abducted, elbow extended, forearm pronated | - dorsiflexion to required position not possible | ☐ 0 |
|---|---|---|
| | - required wrist position possible, no resistance | ☐ 1 |
| | - required position can be maintained against some (slight) resistance | ☐ 2 |

## *Performance*

*Original text*

Wrist stability is tested with the shoulder joint somewhat flexed and/or abducted, elbow joint in the 0° position, the forearm pronated. The examiner may, if needed, support the arm in this position.

*Comments*

Apply resistance only in such cases, where the patient is able to maintain the 15° dorsiflexion against gravity.

## *Scoring*

*Original text*

0: If the patient cannot dorsiflex the wrist in the required position.
1: If dorsiflexion can be performed but no resistance can be taken.
2: The position can be maintained against some (slight) resistance.

## d  Repeated wrist flexion and extension with the elbow fully extended

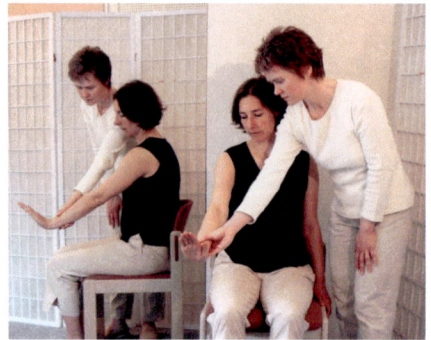 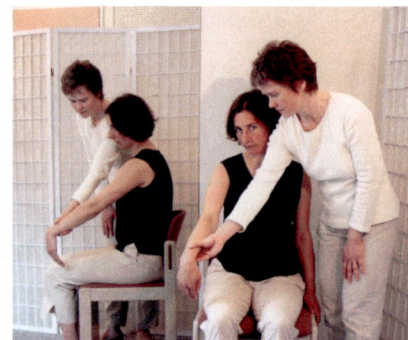

| _d) Repeated max. wrist flexion - extension_<br>shoulder slightly flexed and/or abducted, elbow extended, forearm pronated<br>Score against passive RoM. | - no active repeated movements ☐ 0<br>- active movements smaller than<br>  passive movements ☐ 1<br>- detail is fully and adequately<br>  performed ☐ 2 |
|---|---|

## Performance

*Original text*

Alternate the dorsi- and volar-flexions as previously described but with the shoulder joint somewhat flexed and/or abducted. The elbow fully extended (support if needed)

*Comments*

During wrist extension, the fingers could be somewhat flexed.

*Added specifications*

Do not restrain the forearm. The patient is instructed to keep the forearm in the starting position.

## Scoring

*Original text*

0: Volitional movements do not occur.

1: The patient cannot actively move the wrist joint throughout the total passive range of motion.

2: Each detail is fully and adequately performed.

*Comments*

Repeat the evaluation of passive range of motion in this indicated position in order to decide whether the patient is able to cover the complete range of motion or not. If active RoM covers passive RoM (even when passive RoM is limited), a score of 2 will be allocated. To allocate a score of „1“, the movements have to be repeated in both directions.

Do not mistake release of spasticity for a flicker of active movement

**e      Circumduction of the wrist**

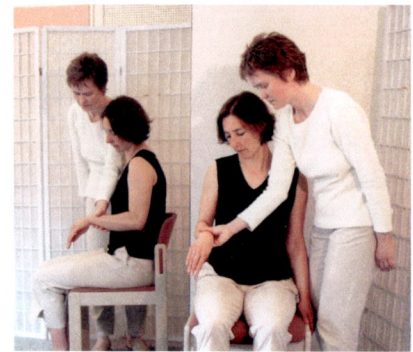 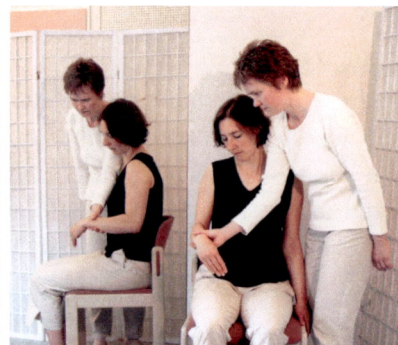

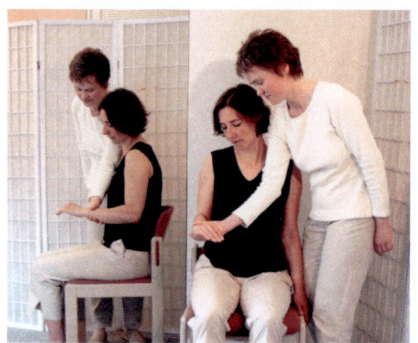

| *e) Circumduction of the wrist* shoulder 0°, elbow 90°. Examiner may provide support for the fore-arm but not restrain it. | - impossible | □ 0 |
|---|---|---|
| | - jerky or incomplete movements | □ 1 |
| | - detail is fully and adequately performed | □ 2 |

## *Performance*

| | |
|---|---|
| *Original text* | *Added specifications* |
| Circumduction of the wrist | The shoulder is kept in 0° (all degrees of freedom) and the elbow in 90°, the examiner may provide support for the forearm, but not restrain it. |

## *Scoring*

*Original text*

0: circumduction cannot be performed

1: jerky motion or incomplete circumduction

2: each detail is fully and adequately performed

## C      Hand

Seven details are evaluated. Of these, five are different types of grasps (with different types of muscular co-contractions). This section of the Fugl-Meyer focuses on the ability of the patient to perform <u>active movements</u>. The examiner may, if necessary, support the elbow in the 90° position; no support may be given for the wrist.

### a      Fingers mass flexion

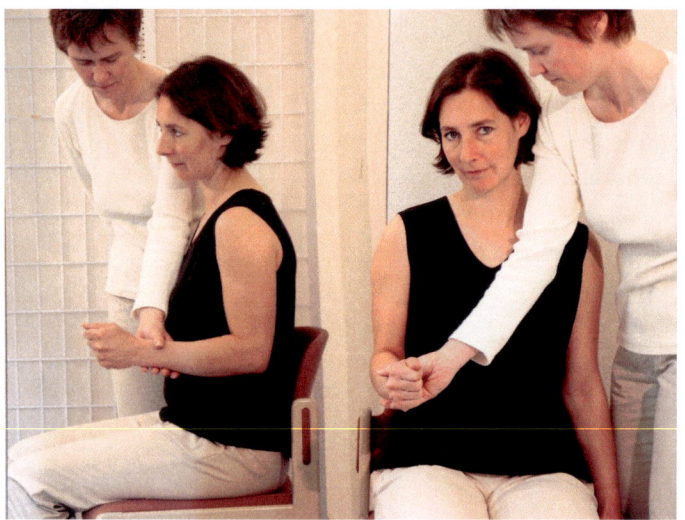

| C. Hand | |
|---|---|
| *a) Flexion of the fingers* | - no flexion                                        ☐ 0 <br> - some, but not full active <br>   flexion                                           ☐ 1 <br> - full active flexion compared <br>   with the unaffected hand        ☐ 2 |

## *Performance*

*Original text*

The patient is instructed to flex his fingers.

*Added specifications*

Starting position of the forearm is neutral with respect to pronation and supination, that of the wrist is neutral where possible. Patient should actively flex fingers from full extension (this position may be facilitated by the assessor).

This test may be linked with the next: fingers mass extension.

## *Scoring*

*Original text*

0: no flexion occurs
1: some, but not full active flexion
2: full active flexion (compared with
   unaffected hand)

**b      Fingers mass extension**

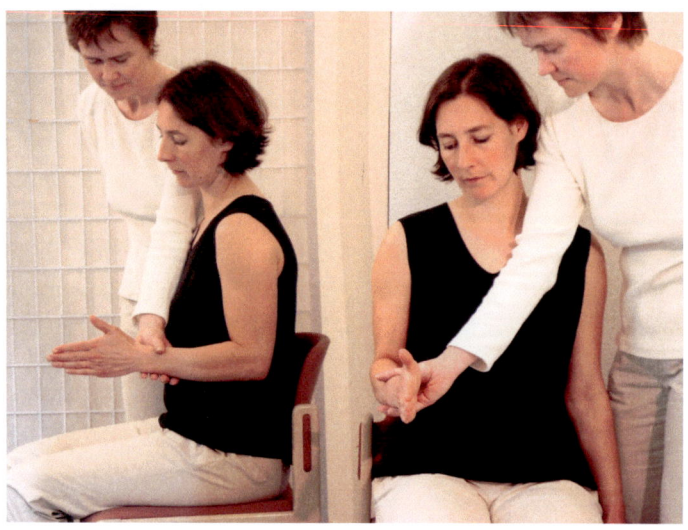

| *b) Extension of the fingers* | - no extension | ☐ 0 |
|---|---|---|
| from the position of full flexion (passive) | - some, but not full ext. or release of an active mass flexion grasp | ☐ 1 |
| | - full active extension, compared with the unaffected hand | ☐ 2 |

## *Performance*

*Original text*

From the position of full active or passive flexion the patient is required to extend all fingers.

*Added specifications*

Starting position of the forearm is neutral with respect to pronation and supination, that of the wrist is neutral where possible. Patient should actively extend fingers from full flexion (this position may be facilitated by the assessor).

## *Scoring*

*Original text*

0:  no extension occurs

1:  some, but not full active extension or release an active mass flexion grasp

2:  full active extension (compared with unaffected hand)

## Grasp tests:

All grasp tests consist of an active (i.e. grasping) and static (i.e. holding against resistance) component which can be clearly distinguished. The required position should be maintained during the tug.

### c      Grasp A

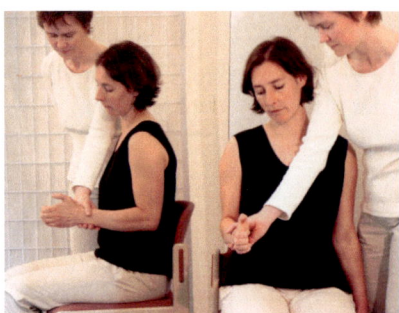 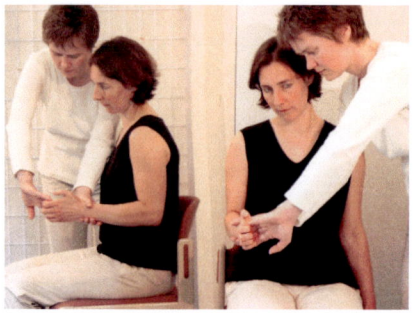

| *c) Grasp A: extension MCP, flexion PIP and DIP*<br>grasp has to be maintained against resistance | - required position not possible ☐ 0<br>- weak grasp ☐ 1<br>- grasp maintained against<br>   relatively great resistance ☐ 2 |
| --- | --- |

MCP:   metacarpophalangeal joints

PIP:   proximal interphalangeal joints

DIP:   distal interphalangeal joints

## Performance

*Original text*

The patient is instructed to extend the metacarpophalangeal joints of digits II-V and flex the proximal and distal interphalangeal joints. The grasp is tested against resistance.

*Added specifications*

Starting position of the forearm is neutral with respect to pronation and supination, that of the wrist is neutral where possible.

Use demonstration and give assistance until the patient understands what is required. However, the patient has to achieve the position actively. Resistance is tested against flexion of the fingers.

## Scoring

*Original text*

0: The required position cannot be acquired.
1: The grasp is weak.
2: The grasp can be maintained against relatively great resistance.

**d      Grasp B**

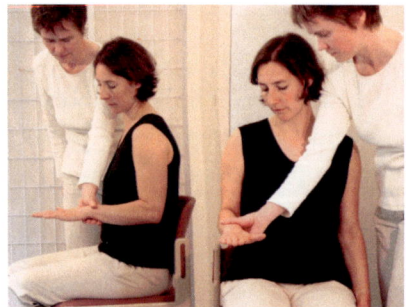 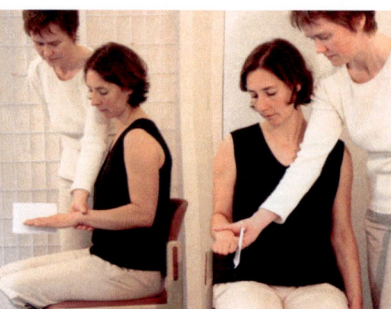

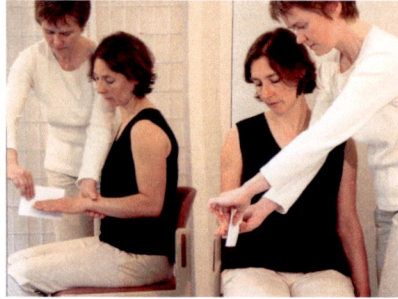

| d) Grasp B: extended index and thumb (holding a sheet with the volar side of the extended thumb and the metacarpale of the index finger against a horizontal tug away from the patient) | - the function as such can not be performed ☐ 0 <br> - scrap of paper kept in place, not against a slight tug ☐ 1 <br> - scrap of paper is held well against a tug ☐ 2 |
|---|---|

## *Performance*

| *Original text* | *Added specifications* |
|---|---|
| The patient should perform a pure thumb adduction, the first carpo-metacarpophalangeal- and interphalangeal joints in the 0° position. | The sheet has to be held with the volar side of the extended thumb and the metacarpale of the index finger and not with the extended or flexed distal phalanges of the index finger. |

The starting position of the wrist is neutral with respect to flexion and extension while the forearm is pronated.

A characteristic of a "tug" is its suddenness. The patient should always be warned of this sudden movement. The direction of the tug should be horizontal, away from the patient.

Object size: ¼ A4 (A6).

## *Scoring*

*Original text*

0: The function as such can not be performed.

1: A scrap of paper interposed between the thumb and the second metacarpals can be kept in place but not against a slight tug.

2: A scrap of paper is held well against a tug.

*Comments*

To allocate a score of „2", there is no relative movement between the paper and the hand.

*Added specifications*

The straightened position of the carpometacarpophalangeal- and interphalangeal joints (0°) of the thumb should be maintained when holding the paper against gravity (score 1 point) and against resistance (score 2 points).

**e      Grasp C**

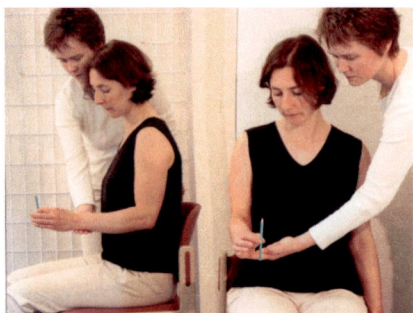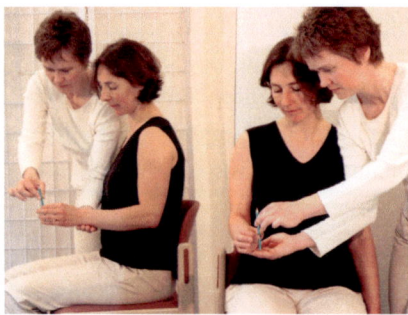

| e) Grasp C: pulpa thumb against the pulpa of the index (holding a pencil with the pulpae of thumb and index finger against an upwards tug) | - the function as such can not be performed ☐ 0 <br> - pencil kept in place, not against a slight tug ☐ 1 <br> - pencil is held well against a tug ☐ 2 |
|---|---|

## *Performance*

| *Original text* | *Comments* |
|---|---|
| The patient opposes his thumb pulpa against the pulpa of the second finger. A pencil is interposed. | The patient should only use the pulpae. The position of the other fingers is not relevant. |
| | The direction of the tug is now upwards, against gravity. The patient is warned of the sudden movement. |

## *Scoring*

| *Original text* | *Comments* |
|---|---|
| 0: The function as such can not be performed. | To allocate a score of „2", there is no relative movement between the pencil and the hand. |
| 1: A pencil interposed between the thumb and the second finger can be kept in place but not against a slight tug. | |
| 2: A pencil is held well against a tug. | |

**f      Grasp D**

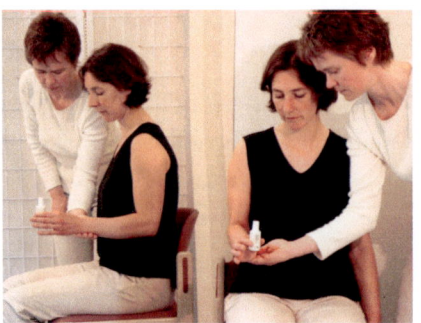 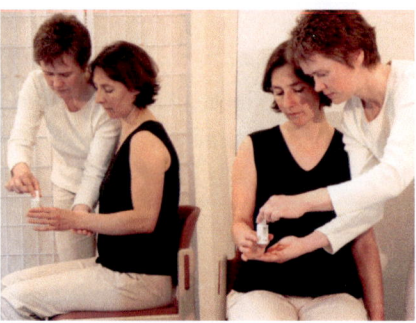

| *f) Grasp D: volar surface of the thumb and index against each other*<br>(holding a cylinder-shaped object against an upwards tug) | - the function as such can not be performed □ 0<br>- cylinder kept in place, not against a slight tug □ 1<br>- cylinder is held well against a tug □ 2 |
|---|---|

## *Performance*

*Original text*

The patient should grasp a cylinder-shaped object (small can), the volar surface of the first and second fingers against each other.

*Comments*

The patient should use the volar surfaces of first and second fingers (i.e. thumb and index finger), the joints are probably slightly bent.

*Added specifications*

The direction of the tug again is upwards, against gravity. The patient is warned of the sudden movement. The object needed could be a Tip-ex® bottle.

## *Scoring*

*Original text*

0: The function as such can not be performed.

1: A small can interposed between the thumb and the second finger can be kept in place but not against a slight tug.

2: A small can is held well against a tug.

*Comments*

To allocate a score of „2", there is no relative movement between the can/bottle and the hand.

**g        Grasp E**

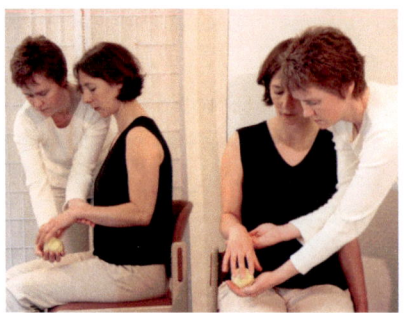 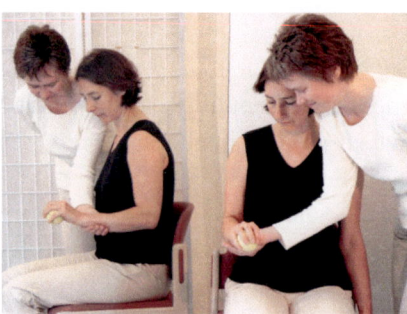

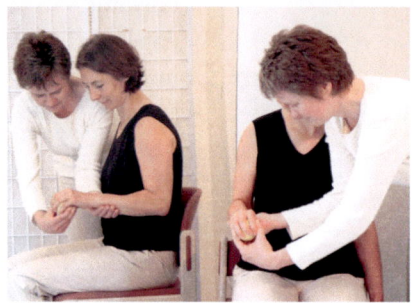

| *g) Grasp E: spherical grasp* (grasping a tennisball and holding it against a downwards tug) | - the function as such can not be performed ☐ 0 <br> - ball grasped, not held against a slight tug ☐ 1 <br> - ball grasped, well held against a tug ☐ 2 |
|---|---|

## Performance

### Original text

A spherical grasp. The patient grasps a tennis ball or is instructed to place his fingers in a position with abduction position of the thumb and abduction flexion of the second, third, fourth and fifth fingers.

### Comments

The patient has to attempt to actively grasp the ball with the forearm pronated, involving active extension and abduction of the fingers. The ball is presented on the palm of the evaluator's hand.

### Added specifications

The patient is warned of the sudden movement, the tug is applied vertically downwards.

## Scoring

### Original text

0: The function as such can not be performed.
1: A tennis ball can be kept in place but not against a slight tug.
2: A tennis ball is held well against a tug.

### Comments

A patient who holds the ball through spasticity or rigidity will achieve a score of 0.
To allocate a score of „2", there is no relative movement between the ball and the hand.

**D      Co-ordination / Speed**

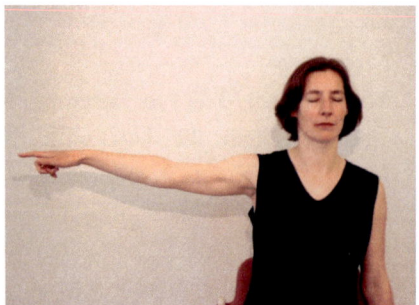 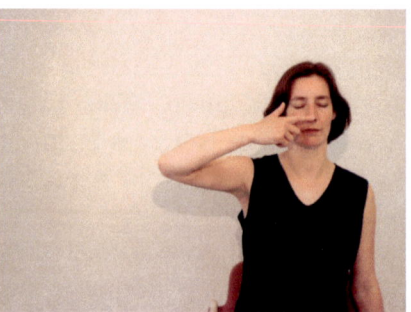

---

### D. Co-ordination/ Speed

*Finger-to-nose test:*
Starting position with the elbow fully extended and the shoulder in 90°abduction

|  | marked | slight | no |
|---|---|---|---|
| a) *Tremor* | ☐ 0 | ☐ 1 | ☐ 2 |

|  | pronounced or unsystematic | slight and systematic | no |
|---|---|---|---|
| *b) Dysmetria* | ☐ 0 | ☐ 1 | ☐ 2 |

| *c) Time* compare time affected to unaffected side | > 6 sec | 2-5 sec | < 2 sec |
|---|---|---|---|
| | ☐ 0 | ☐ 1 | ☐ 2 |
| | time right: | time left: | |
| | sec. | sec. | |

## *Performance*

| *Original text* | *Added specifications* |
|---|---|
| A finger-to-nose test is applied. The patient is instructed to put the tip of his index finger to his nose blindfolded, five times in as rapid succession as he can. | The finger-to-nose test will start with the shoulder in 90° abduction, the elbow extended. No compensating movements of trunk or head are allowed. |

## *Scoring*

*Added specifications*

If the patient cannot assume the starting position, the score will be 0 for all subtests.

## a     **Tremor**

| *Original text* | *Added specifications* |
|---|---|
| 0: marked tremor<br>1: slight tremor<br>2: no tremor | Tremor is interpreted as oscillations <u>during</u> the trajectory from start to endpoint. |

## b     **Dysmetria**

| *Original text* | *Comments* |
|---|---|
| 0: pronounced or unsystematic dysmetria<br>1: slight and systematic dysmetria<br>2: no dysmetria | Dysmetria is interpreted as the error in endpoint destination.<br>A perfect finger-to-nose performance (i.e. score of 2) requires the finger to systematically land in an area of approx. 1 cm$^2$ on the tip of the nose. Unsystematic dysmetria: random errors. Systematic dysmetria: same error (in terms of size and direction) with each performance. |

## c    Time/Speed

*Original text*

The swiftness of motion is com-pared with that of the unaffected side.

0:  the finger-to-nose manoeuvre repeated 5 times is at least 6 seconds slower on the affected side

1:  2-5 seconds slower on the affected side

2:  less than 2 seconds difference

*Added specifications*

The examiner may measure the time with a stopwatch on the videotape or simultaneously during administration of the test. The time is taken from when the patient leaves the full abduction and is stopped when he/she reaches his/her nose for the 5th time.

## Fugl-Meyer Motor Parts: notes for the assessor

| item | independently reach starting position | support possible | compare with passive RoM | repetition |
|---|---|---|---|---|
| **A I** reflex | | | | x |
| **A II b** | | (starting position) | | |
| **A III a** | | (trunk stabilisation) | | |
| **A III b** | | (starting position) | | |
| **A III c** | x | | x | (both directions) |
| **A IV a** | | (starting position) | | |
| **A IV b** | | (starting position) | | |
| **A IV c** | x | | x | (both directions) |
| **A V** | | | | x |
| **B a** | | (elbow) | | |
| **B b** | | (elbow) | x | x |
| **B c** | | (elbow) | | |
| **B d** | | (elbow) | x | x |
| **B e** | | (forearm) | | (one direction) |
| **C a** | | (elbow) | | |
| **C b** | | (elbow and starting position) | | |
| **C c** | | (elbow and resistance) | | |
| **C d** | | (elbow and tug) | | |
| **C e** | | (elbow and tug) | | |
| **C f** | | (elbow and tug) | | |
| **C g** | | (elbow and tug) | | |
| **D** | x | | | (5 times) |

## H   Sensation

### a   Light touch

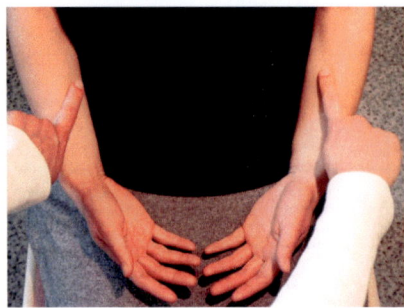 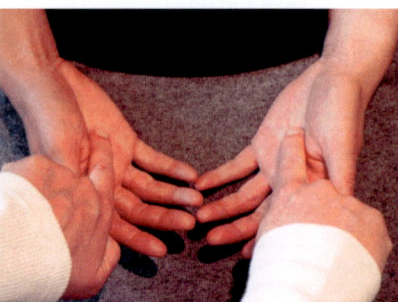

| H. SENSATION | | | |
|---|---|---|---|
| *a) Light touch*<br>Ask the patient whether she/he feels that light touch on both arms and the palmar surface of the hands gave the same qualitative and quantitative impression.<br><br>Score light touch as follows:<br>0:   anaesthesia<br>1:   hypaesthesia, dysaesthesia<br>2:   normaesthesia<br><br>- volar side of the forearm<br>- palmar surface of the hand | <br><br><br><br><br><br><br><br><br><br>☐ 0<br>☐ 0 | <br><br><br><br><br><br><br><br><br><br>☐ 1<br>☐ 1 | <br><br><br><br><br><br><br><br><br><br>☐ 2<br>☐ 2 |

## Performance

*Original text*

The sensation for light touch is roughly estimated. Thus the patient is asked whether he feels that light touch on both arms and the palmar surface of the hands gave the same qualitative and quantitative impression.

*Added specifications*

Apply with the tip of your index finger movements on firstly the volar side of the patient's forearm and secondly on the palmar surface of the hand. The patient is not blindfolded, he/she is asked to concentrate on the sensations. Apply as many stimuli as needed to score this item.

Ask the patient whether she/he feels the touch, and whether there is a difference compared with the other side concerning the quality or quantity. Ask: Do you feel my finger touching you? Is there any difference between the right and the left side?

## Scoring

*Original text*

0: anaesthesia
1: hypaesthesia/dysaesthesia
2: normaesthesia

*Added specifications*

Score „0", if the patient does not feel a single stimulus

Score „1", if the patient describes a difference between left and right sides in terms of quality or quantity of sensation.

Score „2" when she/he feels each light touch without difference between the limbs.

**b    Position sense**

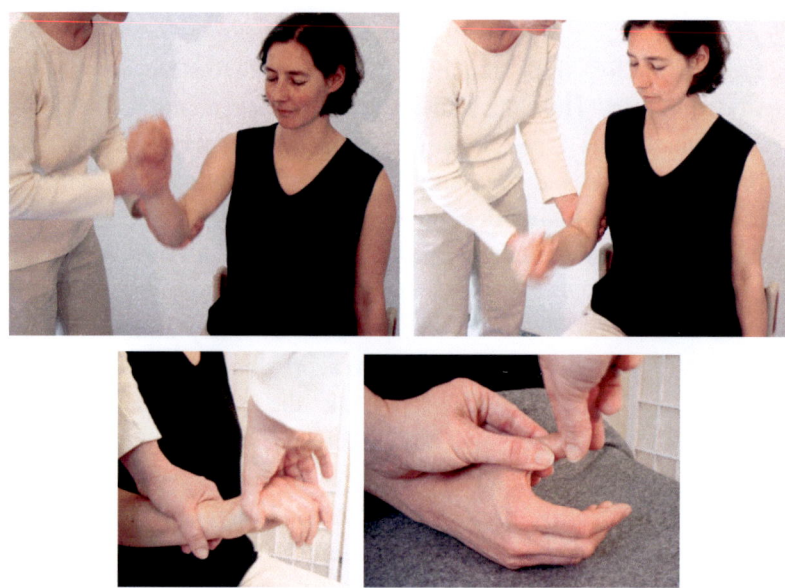

| b) Position sense of the joints | | | |
|---|---|---|---|
| Patient blindfolded. Score position sense of the joints as follows:<br>0:  absence of sensation<br>1:  considerable difference compared with the joint on the unaffected side, but at least ¾ of the answers correct<br>2:  all answers correct, little or no difference comparing unaffected with affected limb | | | |
| - glenohumeral joint | ☐ 0 | ☐ 1 | ☐ 2 |
| - elbow | ☐ 0 | ☐ 1 | ☐ 2 |
| - wrist | ☐ 0 | ☐ 1 | ☐ 2 |
| - thumb (interphalangeal joint) | ☐ 0 | ☐ 1 | ☐ 2 |

## *Performance*

### *Original text*

The position sense of the joints is tested for the thumb (interphalangeal joint), the wrist, the elbow and the glenohumeral joint. Very small alterations in the position are accomplished by the examiner who also takes care to place his fingers and his hand so that other qualities of sensation than the position sense of the joints do not lead the patients to conclusions. The examiner should also take care to avoid excitation of the primary ending when altering the joint position, as the patient may detect changes in position through I a gamma-fibres. The patient is blindfolded. Both sides are tested, starting with non-affected side. The affected side is tested after the latter has been completed. The assessor demonstrates and gives an example of what is expected of the patient. Movements are small and end RoM is avoided. The patient indicates verbally to the assessor in which direction the joint is moved. If this is not possible, the patient is asked to imitate the movement with the non-affected side. Skin contact is minimised to avoid giving the patient information about the change in position through the skin receptors. Each joint is tested 4 times in the direction of flexion and extension.

### *Added specifications*

Apply the small movements each in a flexion-extension direction throughout the submaximum of the passive range of motion.

Elbow:
- shoulder neutral in all planes
- forearm in midposition pronation/ supination

Wrist:
- shoulder neutral in all planes
- elbow 90° flexion
- forearm pronated (palm of hand facing down if possible)
- assessor stabilises forearm and moves hand, handling the latter by its radial and ulnar borders

Thumb:
- the supinated arm is lying in the patient's lap
- the thumb is handled from the lateral sides
- the assessor stabilises the proximal phalanx of the thumb and moves the distal phalanx

## Scoring

### Original text

0: absence of sensation

1: considerable difference in sensation compared with the joint on the unaffected side, but at least ¾ of the answers correct

2: all answers correct, little or no difference comparing unaffected with affected limb

## J    Passive Joint Motion

| J. PASSIVE JOINT MOTION / JOINT PAIN | | | |
|---|---|---|---|
| a) Passive joint motion<br>Score passive joint motion as follows:<br>0:  only few degrees of RoM<br>1:  decreased passive RoM<br>2:  normal passive RoM | | | |
| Shoulder    flexion | ☐ 0 | ☐ 1 | ☐ 2 |
| abduction to 90 ° | ☐ 0 | ☐ 1 | ☐ 2 |
| outw. rotation | ☐ 0 | ☐ 1 | ☐ 2 |
| inw. rotation | ☐ 0 | ☐ 1 | ☐ 2 |
| Elbow    flexion | ☐ 0 | ☐ 1 | ☐ 2 |
| extension | ☐ 0 | ☐ 1 | ☐ 2 |
| Forearm    pronation | ☐ 0 | ☐ 1 | ☐ 2 |
| supination | ☐ 0 | ☐ 1 | ☐ 2 |
| Wrist    flexion | ☐ 0 | ☐ 1 | ☐ 2 |
| extension | ☐ 0 | ☐ 1 | ☐ 2 |
| Fingers    flexion | ☐ 0 | ☐ 1 | ☐ 2 |
| extension | ☐ 0 | ☐ 1 | ☐ 2 |

## *Performance*

### *Original text*

Evaluation of passive joint motion and occurrence of joint pain during and at the end of the passive motion of a joint performed for most joints of the affected limbs. Joint motion is compared with the non-affected extremity. It may often be advantageous to evaluate joint motion and joint pain before assessing the motor function, as dysfunction of a joint per se should be disregarded when evaluating the motor function.

As it is felt that the examiner should be able to evaluate joint motion/joint pain on a bedridden patient, the abduction of the shoulder is performed only to 90° .

## Comments

Actually, it is recommended that this section be assessed at the beginning of the Fugl-Meyer test. The patient is seated.

Each movement is tested to the full and the patient is asked to indicate if there is any pain.

Added specifications:

Shoulder: Abduction to 90°:

· examiner ensures patient can not compensate with elevation of the shoulder girdle.

· elbow is flexed for ease of handling

Shoulder: Outward rotation:

· shoulder: neutral in all planes

· elbow: 90° flexion

Shoulder: Inward rotation:

· shoulder: neutral in all planes

· elbow: 90° flexion

· Examiner moves patient's hand towards chest

Elbow: Flexion and extension:

· shoulder: neutral in all planes

· elbow: mid position pronation-supination

Pronation-Supination:

· shoulder and elbow: 90° flexion

Wrist: Flexion and extension:

· shoulder: neutral in all planes

· elbow: 90° flexion, pronation (hand-palm facing down)

Fingers: Flexion and extension:

· shoulder: neutral in all planes

· elbow: 90° flexion, midposition pronation/ supination.

## *Scoring*

### *Original text*

0: only a few degrees of range-of-motion

1: decreased passive range-of-motion

2: normal passive range-of-motion

## J   Joint Pain

| J.  PASSIVE  JOINT  MOTION / JOINT PAIN | | | |
|---|---|---|---|
| *b) Joint pain*<br>Score  occurrence  of  joint  pain  as follows:<br>0:  pronounced  pain  during  all  the movement  or  very  marked  pain  at the  end  of  the  actual  range  of motion<br>1:  some pain<br>2:  no pain | | | |
| Shoulder      flexion | ☐ 0 | ☐ 1 | ☐ 2 |
|                      abduction to 90 ° | ☐ 0 | ☐ 1 | ☐ 2 |
|                      outw. rotation | ☐ 0 | ☐ 1 | ☐ 2 |
|                      inw. rotation | ☐ 0 | ☐ 1 | ☐ 2 |
| Elbow          flexion | ☐ 0 | ☐ 1 | ☐ 2 |
|                      extension | ☐ 0 | ☐ 1 | ☐ 2 |
| Forearm      pronation | ☐ 0 | ☐ 1 | ☐ 2 |
|                      supination | ☐ 0 | ☐ 1 | ☐ 2 |
| Wrist          flexion | ☐ 0 | ☐ 1 | ☐ 2 |
|                      extension | ☐ 0 | ☐ 1 | ☐ 2 |
| Fingers       flexion | ☐ 0 | ☐ 1 | ☐ 2 |
|                      extension | ☐ 0 | ☐ 1 | ☐ 2 |

***Performance***

*Added specifications*
The patient is asked to indicate if there is any pain during the passive movements.

***Scoring occurrence of joint pain***

*Original text*

0: pronounced pain during all the movement or very marked pain at the end of the actual range of motion

1: some pain

2: no pain

*Added specifications*
Score „0", when patient interrupts the assessment because of pain, when very marked pain occurs at the end of the actual range of motion or when there is pronounced pain during the entire RoM.

Score „1", when patient allows full RoM but also indicates pain.

# 5.3. Manual for the Action Research Arm test

## 5.3.1. General remarks

Interpretation of the Action Research Arm Test and the material

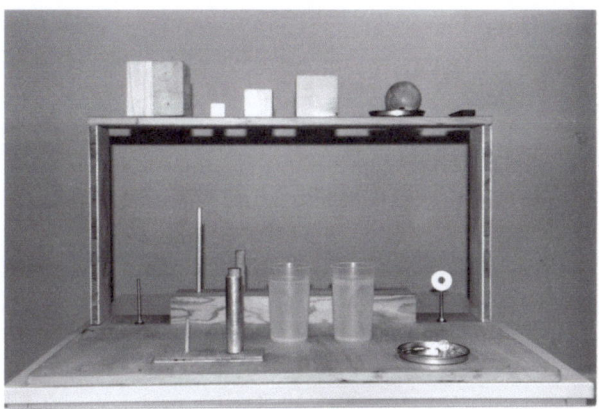

The ARAT, developed by Lyle (1981), is based on the Upper Extremity Function Test published by Carroll (1965). Lyle omitted several items and ordered the tasks in four subtests. His description of the objects and starting positions was not as precise as the details provided by Carroll. Although Lyle indicated the deviations from the original version, he also writes: „An attempt was made to duplicate as closely as possible the test materials used by Carroll in his earlier study, given certain constraints on the local availability of materials, and incorporating some simplification." (p. 486)

Therefore, the information concerning material and test performance has to be inferred in some cases. This manual presents the Action Research Arm Test designed by Lyle with additional instructions based on Carroll´s publication where necessary.

## Construction of the test materials

Since the ARAT is not commercially available, it needs to be purpose-built. The basic apparatus consists of a wooden platform (72 x 44 cm) with a shelf placed on a standard height table (appr. 75 cm). The plank is not fixed since it needs to be turned according to the side being assessed (subtest "grip"). We suggest a small mobile platform as starting position for the metal tubes since this is easier to handle than fixed starting positions which would have to be constructed for both limbs. The target point for the washer (subtest "grip") has to be fixed on a certain place, for each side separately. All other objects are mobile and have to be placed on the platform according to the description for each test item.

Construction of the test material should be based on the information that has been provided in chapter 3.2.2.

## General performance and scoring

Wherever possible, the patient is seated on an ordinary chair (height 44 cm +/- 2 cm) without armrests - rarely in his own wheelchair - in front of the table. He/she may be as close to the table as he/she finds necessary to perform the tests and may move along the table if this is helpful. The patient is not allowed to rise from the chair during the test, although he or she may lean to one side. Each hand is tested separately, firstly with the non or less affected side. The tester explains the tests until the patient clearly understands what is expected. With some patients it may be necessary to demonstrate each test separately prior to the actual item.

The starting position for each task (except subtest Gross Movement) is with the tested arm placed on the wooden platform. Test items are placed appropriately for the side being tested and are presented one at a time. Apart from this requirement, there is no precise starting and destination location for any of the test items.

The patient is allowed to rest between the tasks. He/she does not receive therapeutical interventions e.g. to reduce elevated muscle tone.

The patient is not encouraged to practice several times. However, when the patient performs one practice trial before the actual test, you will score the best performance and not automatically the „actual test".

Lyle introduced performance and scoring guidelines as follows (Lyle; 1981:491):

*The Action Research Arm test „is divided into 4 subtests (Grasp, Grip, Pinch, Gross Movement.). Items within each subtest are ordered in such a way that if the patient scores „3" on item one, (the most difficult) he would almost certainly score „3" on all other items in that subtest, involving the same side. Thus, if a score of „3" is obtained on item one, the patient is being credited with having scored „3" on all items of that subtest for that (left or right) side, without having to be tested on the remaining subtest items.*

*If the patient scores less than „3" on item one, then item two is administered. Item two is the easiest item in each subtest, and if the patient scores „0" then he is unlikely to achieve a score above zero on any item in the subtest for that side (left or right) on which a zero score was obtained. Thus he is credited with a zero subtest total score for that side, and you should move to the next subtest.*

*If however, the patient scores less than „3" on item one and more than zero on item two, all items in the Subtest must be administered.*

*This sounds complicated to explain, but it is easy in practice. The result is an average saving of 50% in testing time."*

## Scoring instructions for examiner

There are four grades for each test of the total evaluation:

Grade 3:     The test is performed normally.

Grade 2:     Patient completes test, but takes abnormally long time or has great difficulty. The performance is slowly or very clumsily. Completion of the test consists of placing the test item in the correct position, pouring the water, placing the hand in the indicated position.

Grade 1:     The patient completes parts of the test. The grade is given when the patient is able to pick up or lift the item from the table or from its slot, but is unable to place the object in its correct position. In item "pour water from glass to glass", the patient is able to pick up the glass but unable to pour water into its proper receptacle.

Grade 0:     The patient is unable to perform any part of the test. Pushing objects out of their slots or around the table is graded 0.

### *Added specifications*

Scoring is not really based on a comparison of both sides; however, in patients with unilateral impairment, the non-affected side might help the rater by observing normal behaviour. To reduce one point from "performs test normally", the patient has to show great difficulties and not only a small difference in duration of the movement compared with the other side. There is no quantitative time limit for performing the test. For patients with bilateral impairment comparing the two sides is not helpful to determine whether behaviour on either side is normal. When comparing left and right side when both sides are affected, compare with the norm of non-impaired function.

## 5.3.2. How to perform and score the Action Research Arm test - specific remarks

A.     Subtest Grasp

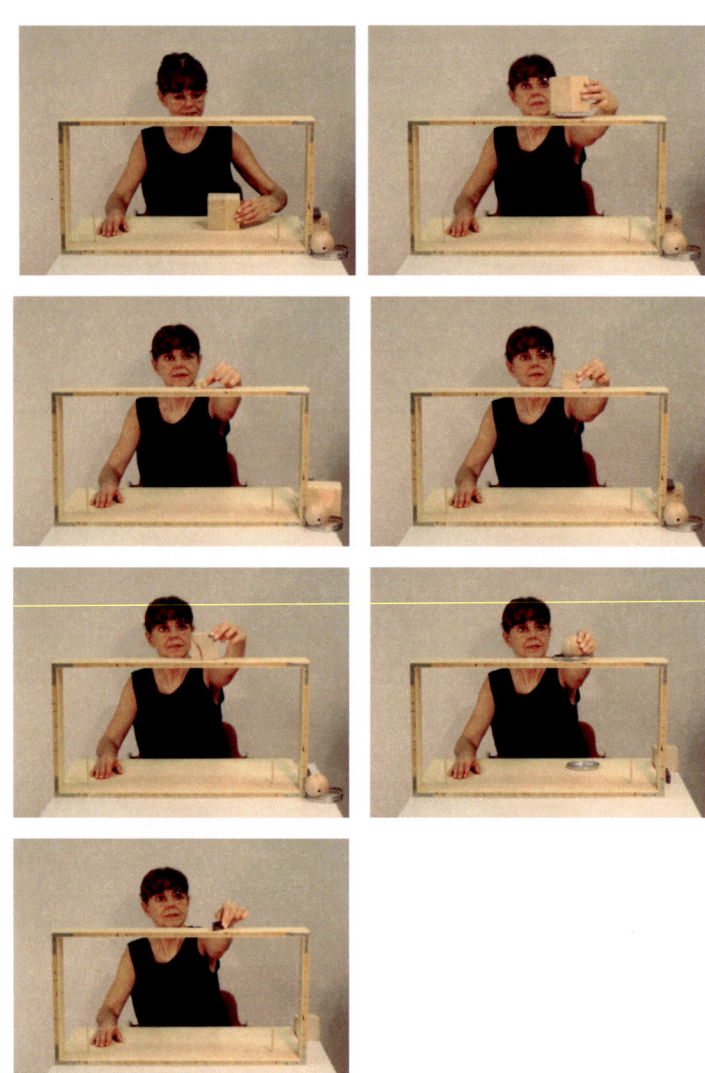

Order: from left to right and from top to bottom

*Performance*

The items have to be lifted from the trolley surface to the shelf above it. All items must first be grasped by open-handed grasp and secondly raised to the shelf (ca. 30cm above the table). The test items are placed appropriately for the side being tested. Once the patient has completed a task, the item is taken away by the examiner. The examiner presents the objects one at a time in the following order: block 10 cm, block 2.5 cm, block 5 cm, block 7.5 cm, ball 7.5 cm, stone (placed on its long side). The stone is positioned on its narrow, long side and has to be grasped by lateral prehension.

*Scoring*

In cases where the patient cannot grasp the item, test item is aborted and the score is 0.

A score of 1 is assigned if the patient can grasp the item and lift it from the table, but cannot reach the shelf because the necessary upper arm and shoulder function has been impaired.

In cases where a patient has placed and released the object, the task is finished and the patient obtains the score for his/her performance to the endpoint of the task (pick->transport->place ->release).

If the object cannot be released at the endpoint, a score of less than 3 is appropriate.

If a patient releases the object at the end position but knocks it over on the way down, he/she should not be penalised.

| GRASP | | Evaluation | |
| --- | --- | --- | --- |
| | | **Left** | **Right** |
| 1 | Woodblock 10 cm (If score = 3, total = 18 and go to Grip) | | |
| 2 | Woodblock 2.5 cm (If score = 0, total = 0 and go to Grip) | | |
| 3 | Woodblock 5 cm | | |
| 4 | Woodblock 7.5 cm | | |
| 5 | Cricketball 7.5 cm diameter | | |
| 6 | Stone 10 x 2.5 x 1 cm | | |
| **SUBTOTAL** *Grasp* | | /18 | /18 |

## B.    Subtest Grip

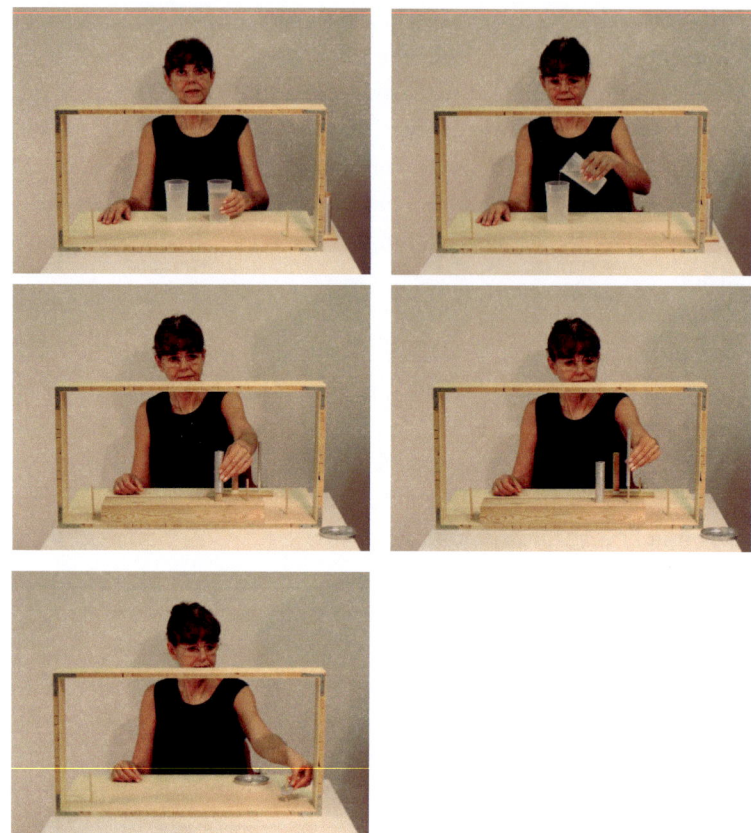

Order: from left to right and from top to bottom

Subtest Grip shares elements in common with Grasp, except that some degree of mobility of the wrist is required, including flexion/extension and pronation/supination.

*Performance*

1. Pour water from glass to glass. The tumblers are placed in front of the patient, on either side of the patient's midline. The tumblers stand close together, at no fixed distance, but do not touch. The patient is allowed to stabilise the second tumbler with the other hand in a vertical position, the assessor can also stabilise the second tumbler instead of the patient.

2. & 3. The two tubes of different sizes (2.25 cm x 11.5 cm; 1.0 cm x 16 cm), which are placed over the vertical peg close to the patient, are to be moved and placed over the vertical peg, positioned further forward (appr. 30 cm) on the plank.

4. the patient also has to pick up an iron washer, which is placed in a tin lid, and let it slide down a vertical bolt, 30 cm further on the surface.

*Scoring*

1. Performance has to involve pronation of the forearm; if the patient merely laterally bends the trunk without pronating the forearm (even if the water is poured into the other glass) the task is not completed-> score =1.

| GRIP | | Evaluation | |
|---|---|---|---|
| | | **Left** | **Right** |
| 1 | Pour water from glass to glass (pronation) (If score = 3, total = 12 and go to Pinch) | | |
| 2 | Tube 2.25 cm (If score = 0, total = 0 and go to Pinch) | | |
| 3 | Tube 1 cm | | |
| 4 | Washer over bolt | | |
| SUBTOTAL *Grip* | | /12 | /12 |

## C.    Subtest Pinch

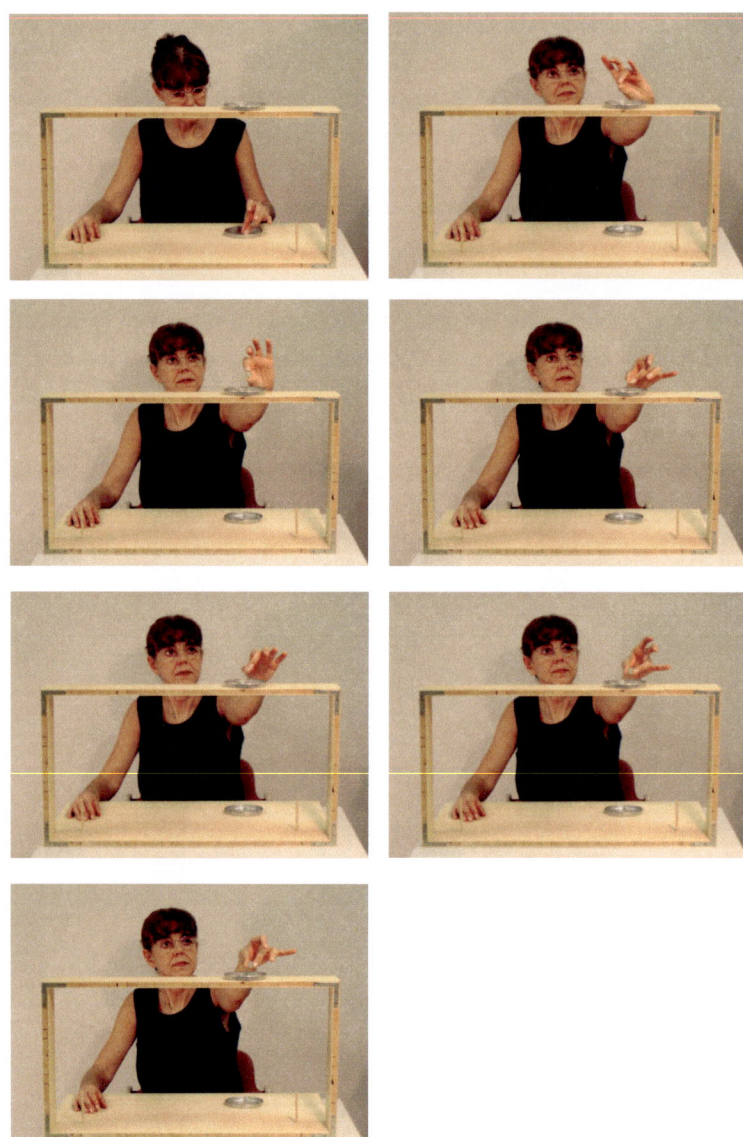

Order: from left to right and from top to bottom

Subtest Pinch is a test of finger-thumb opposition, incorporated within a test of upper arm and shoulder function.

*Performance*

There is a tray (tobacco tin lid) with a rim to contain the ball bearing or the marble, respectively. The spheres are to be moved one by one to a similar tray on the shelf. The patient has to grasp one by one the ball-bearings and the marble in a strict order:

| PINCH | | Evaluation | |
|---|---|---|---|
| | | **Left** | **Right** |
| 1 | Ball bearing, 6 mm, thumb and ring finger (If score = 3, total = 18 and go to Gross movement) | | |
| 2 | Marble, 1.5 cm, thumb and index finger (If score = 0, total = 0 and go to Gross movement) | | |
| 3 | Ball bearing thumb and middle finger | | |
| 4 | Ball bearing thumb and index finger | | |
| 5 | Marble thumb and ring finger | | |
| 6 | Marble thumb and middle finger | | |
| **SUBTOTAL** *Pinch* | | /18 | /18 |

## D.    Subtest Gross Movement

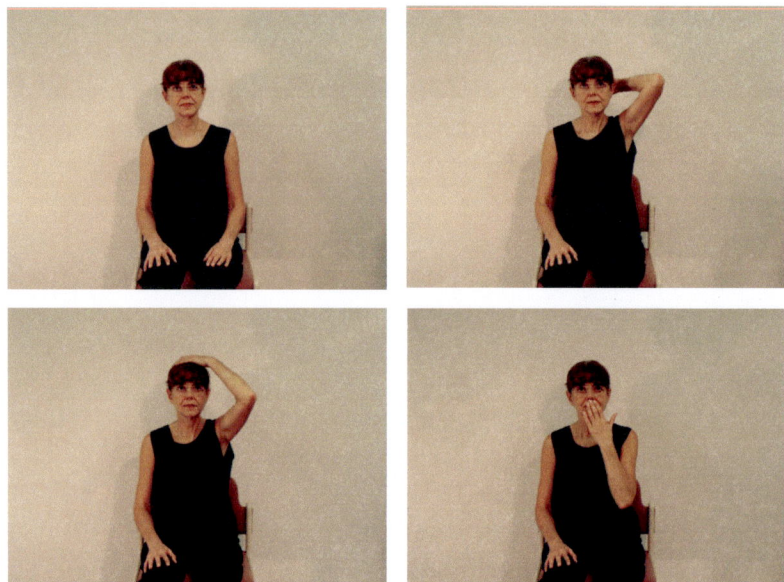

Order: from left to right and from top to bottom;
left upper photo denotes the starting position

Subtest gross movement requires preservation of some degree of upper arm and shoulder function.

*Performance*
1. Place hand behind head
2. Place hand on top of head
3. Hand to mouth

The starting position of the arm is either lying in the patient's lap or at the patient's side. Items 1 & 2 are administered only once. For item 1, the hand is to be placed behind the <u>head</u>, not the neck. For item 2, place hand on top of head, not on the forehead.

If the patient cannot perform the first item, the test will be aborted.

The patient needs to remain in an upright posture, to allow a fair evaluation of the function of the shoulder joint. The patient needs to be carefully instructed and the task needs to be demonstrated, to ensure that the patient avoids compensatory strategies.

*Scoring*

If the head is bent down to facilitate task, the task is not complete -> score =1.

If the head is bent down, after which extension of neck facilitates reaching the correct end position -> score =2 (some compensatory movement with the trunk is allowed throughout the test).

| GROSS MOVEMENT | | **Evaluation** | |
|---|---|---|---|
| | | **Left** | **Right** |
| 1 | Place hand behind head (If score = 3, total = 9 and finish; if score = 0, total = 0 and finish) | | |
| 2 | Place hand on top of head | | |
| 3 | Hand to mouth | | |
| **SUBTOTAL** *Gross movement* | | /9 | /9 |

Total score

| Total score (all subtests) | /57 | /57 |
|---|---|---|

## 5.4. Manual for the Box and Block test

### 5.4.1. Specific remarks

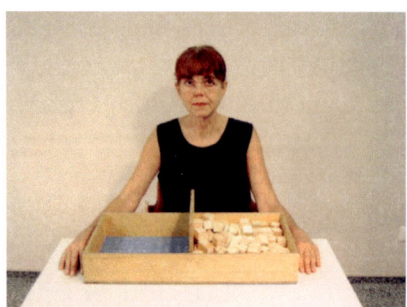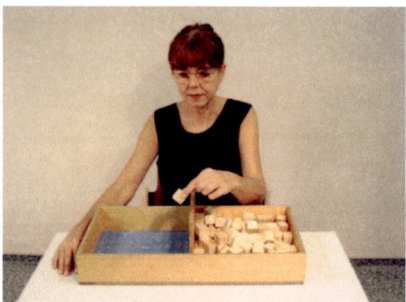

Instructions to the patient

Referring to Mathiowetz et al., 1985:388, the following directions are read to the subject:

*„I want to see how quickly you can pick up one block at a time with your right (or left) hand [the examiner points to the hand]. Carry it to the other side of the box and drop it. Make sure your fingertips cross the partition. Watch me while I show you how."*

The examiner then transports three cubes over the partition in the same direction she or he wants the subject to move them. After a demonstration the examiner says the following.

*„If you pick up two blocks at a time, they will count as one. If you drop one on the floor or table after you have carried it across, it will still be counted, so do not waste time picking it up. If you toss the blocks without crossing the partition, they will not be counted. Before you start, you will have a chance to practice for 15 seconds. Do you have any questions? Place your hands on the sides of the box. When it is time to start, I will say ' ready ' and then ' go '."*

The stopwatch is started at the word *"go"*. When the 15 seconds have passed, the examiner says *"stop"*. If mistakes are made during the practice period, they are corrected before the actual testing begins. On completion of the practice period, the transported cubes are returned to the compartment. The examiner mixes the cubes to assure random distribution.

The examiner continues with the following directions:

*"This will be the actual test. The instructions are the same. Work as quickly as you can. Ready. [The examiner waits 3 seconds.] Go. [After 1 minute.] Stop.*
*[Counting is recorded as described.] Now you are to do the same thing with your left (or right) hand. First you can practice. Put your hands on the sides of the box as before. Pick up one block at a time with your hand, and drop it on the other side of the box. Ready. [The examiner waits 3 seconds] Go. [After 15 seconds] Stop."*

The transported blocks are returned to the compartment as described above.

*"This will be the actual test. The instructions are the same. Work as quickly as you can. Ready. [The examiner waits 3 seconds] Go. [After 1 minute] Stop."*

## Performance and Scoring

### *Performance*

*Original text*

The test box is placed lengthways along the edge of a standard-height table. Each subject is seated on a standard-height chair facing the box. The 150 cubes are in the compartment of the test box on the side where the subjects non-affected (dominant) hand is. The examiner sits facing the subject so she or he can view the blocks being transported. A 15-second trial period precedes the testing. Immediately before testing begins, the subject places their hands on the sides of the box. On signal, the subject grasps one block at a time with the non-affected (dominant) hand, transports the block over the partition, and releases it into the opposite compartment. By use of a digital stop watch the subject is stopped after one minute. The procedure is then repeated with the affected (non-dominant) hand.

*Comments*

The midline of the box should be placed in the patient's midline. The blocks should be thrown into the box randomly and then evenly spread out. The examiner should not encourage the patient to „think of a strategy" or to count during the test period.

*Added specifications*

The test does not require a specific grasp, any grasp is accepted, so long as only 1 block is transported at a time. The hands of the patient are placed to the sides of the box as starting position. Once over the partition, the block is to be dropped - not to be placed.

Do not allow the patient to shuffle the blocks during the test. Take care that each block crosses the partition as well as the finger tips of the patient.

## *Scoring*

*Original text*

The score is the number of blocks carried from one compartment to the other in one minute. If the subject transports two or more blocks at the same time, this is noted and the number is subtracted from the total. If the patient tosses the blocks without crossing the partition, they will not be counted. No penalty is made if the subjects transport any blocks across the partition and the blocks bounce from the box to the floor or table.

*Added specifications:*

The evaluator should pay attention to (either simultaneously or via videotape scoring) on various invalid performances. Several performance behaviours do not produce valid numbers of trans-ported blocks, e.g. transporting a block in front of the partition is not valid. Additionally to the above mentioned guidelines, the patient is not allowed to shuffle blocks into an easier position. Blocks are randomly distributed at the start of the test only.

| | Left | Right |
|---|---|---|
| **Score** | | |

# 6. References

Adams, R.J., Mador, K., Sethi, K.D., Grotta, J.C., Thompson, D.S. (1987) Graded neurological scale for use in acute hemispheric stroke treatment protocols. Stroke; 18:665-669

Adams S.A., Ashburn A., Pickering R.M., Taylor D. (1997a) The scalability of the Rivermead Motor Assessment in acute stroke patients. Clinical Rehabilitation; 11:42-51

Adams S.A., Ashburn A., Pickering R.M., Taylor D. (1997b) The scalability of the Rivermead Motor Assessment in nonacute stroke patients. Clinical Rehabilitation; 11:52-59

Adams, S.A. The Rivermead Motor Assessment for stroke. In: Harrison, M. ed. Physiotherapy in stroke management. Edinburgh: Churchill Livingstone, 1995

Agnew, P.J., Maas, F. (1982) Hand function related to age and sex. Arch Phys Med Rehabil; 63:269-271

Agre, J.C., Magness, J.L., Hull, S.Z., Wright, K.C., Baxter, T.L., Patterson, R., Stradel, L. (1987) Strength testing with a portable dynamometer: reliability for upper and lower extremities. Arch Phys Med Rehabil; 68:454-458

Alderman, E. (1949) Comparison of one-trial and three-trial Purdue Pegboard norms. Occupations; 27:251-2

American Academy of Orthopaedic Surgeons: Joint motion: Method of measuring and recording, 1965

American Guidance Service: Minnesota Rate of Manipulation Test Examiner's Manual. Circle Pines, Minnesota: AGS, 1969

Annett, M., Kilshaw, D. (1983) Right and left hand skill. Br J Psychol; 74:269-283

Arsenault, B., Dutil, E., Lambert, J., Corriveau, H., Guarna, F., Drouin, G. (1988) An evaluation of the hemiplegic subject based on the Bobath approach. Part 3: A validation study. Scand J Rehabil Med; 20:13-16

Ashburn, A. (1982) A physical assessment for stroke patients. Physiotherapy; 68:109-113

Ashworth, B. (1964) Preliminary trial of carisoprodol in multiple sclerosis. Practioner; 192:540-542

Ayre, R., Mockett, S. (2000) Reliability of the Motor Club Assessment (abstract). Physiotherapy; 86:150

Badke, M.B., Duncan, P.W. (1983) Patterns of rapid motor responses during postural adjustments, when standing, in healthy subjects and hemiplegic patients. Phys Ther; 63:13-20

Bard, G., Hirschberg, G.G. (1965) Recovery of voluntary motion in upper extremity following hemiplegia. Arch Phys Med Rehabil; 567-572

Bass, B.M., Stucki, R.E. (1951) A note on a modified Purdue Pegboard. Journal of Applied Psychology; 35:312-13

Bennett, G.K.: Hand Tool Dexterity Test Manual. New York: Harcourt Brace Jovanovich, 1981

Berglund, K., Fugl-Meyer, A.R. (1986) Upper extremity function in hemiplegia. A cross-validation study of two assessment methods. Scand J Rehab Med; 18:155-157

Bernspang, B., Fisher, A.G. (1995) Differences between persons with right or left cerebral vascular accident on the assessment of motor and process skills. Arch Phys Med Rehabil; 76:1144-51

Bohannon, R.W., Andrews, A.W. (1987) Interrater reliability of hand-held dynamometry. Physical Therapy; 67:931-3

Bohannon, R.W., Smith, M.B. (1987) Interrater reliability of a modified Ashworth scale of muscle spasticity. Physical Therapy; 67:206-207

Boissy, P., Bourbonnais, D., Carlotti, M.M., Gravel, D., Arsenault, B.A. (1999) Maximal grip force in chronic subjects and its relationship to global upper extremity function. Clinical Rehabilitation; 13:354-362

Bravo, G., Potvin, L. (1991) Estimating the reliability of continuos measures with Cronbach's alpha or the intraclass correlation coefficient: towards the integration of two traditions. J Clin Epidemiol; 44:381-390

Brunnström, S. (1966) Motor testing procedures in hemiplegia. J Am Phys Ther Ass; 46:357

Brunnström, S. Movement therapy in hemiplegia. A neurophysiological approach. Harper & Row, Hagerstown, 1970

Buddenberg, L.A., Davis, C. (2000) Test-retest reliability of the Purdue Pegboard test. American Journal for Occupational Therapy; 55:555-558

Carr, J.H., Shepherd, R.B., Nordholm, L., Lynne D. (1985) Investigation of a new motor assessment scale for stroke patients. Phy Ther; 65:175-180

Carroll, D. (1965) A Quantitative Test of Upper Extremity Function. Journal of Chronic Disease; 18:479-491

Chae J, Labatia I, Yang G. (2003) Upper limb motor function in hemiparesis: concurrent validity of the Arm Motor Ability test. *Am J Phys Med Rehabil*; 82: 1-8

Clopton, N., Schafer, S., Clopton, J.R., Winer, J-L. (1984) Examinee position and performance on the Minnesota Rate of Manipulation Test. Journal of Rehabilitation, Jan/Feb/March, 46-48

Cohen, J.A., Fisher, J.S., Bolibrush, D.M., Jak, A.K., Kniker, J.E., Mertz, L.A., Skaramagas, T.T., Cutter, G.R. (2000) Intrarater and interrater reliability of the MS functional composite outcome measure. Neurology; 54:802-806

Collen, F.M., Wade, D.T., Bradshaw, C.M. (1990) Mobility after stroke: reliability of measures of impairment and disability. International Disability Studies; 12:6-9

Collen, F.M., Wade, D.T., Robb, G.F., Bradshaw, C.M. (1991) The Rivermead Mobility Index: a further development of the Rivermead Motor Assessment. Int Disabil Stud; 13:50-54

Collin, C., Wade, D. (1990) Assessing motor impairment after stroke: a pilot reliability study. Journal of Neurology, Neurosurgery, and Psychiatry; 53:576-579

Costa, L.D., Vaughan, H.G., Jr., Levita, E., Farber, N. (1963) Purdue Pegboard as a predictor of the presence and laterality of cerebral lesions. Journal of Consulting Psycholgy; 27:133-37

Crow, J.L., Lincoln, N.B., Nouri, F.M. and W. de Weerdt (1989) The effectiveness of EMG biofeedback in the treatment of arm function after stroke. International Disability Studies; 11:155-60

De Souza, L.H., Langton Hewer, R., Lynn, P.A., Miller, S., Reed, G.A.L. (1980b) Recovery of arm control in hemiplegic stroke patients. 2. Comparison of arm function tests and pursuit tracking in relation to clinical recovery. Int Rehab Med; 2:10-16

De Souza, L.H., Langton Hewer, R., Miller, S. (1980a) Assessment of recovery of arm control in hemiplegic stroke patients. 1. Arm function tests. International Rehabilitation Medicine; 2:3-9

De Weerdt, W.J.G., Harrison, M.A. (1985) Measuring recovery of arm-hand-function in stroke patients: A comparison of the Brunnstrom-Fugl-Meyer test and Action Research Arm test. Physiotherapy Canada; 37:65-70

Dean, C., Mackey, F. (1992) Motor Assessment Scale scores as a measure of rehabilitation outcome following stroke. Aust J Physiother; 38:31-35

Demeurisse, G., Demol, O., Robaye, E. (1980) Motor evaluation in vascular hemiplegia. European Neurology; 19:382-9

Desrosiers, J, Bravo, G, Hébert, R, Dutil, E, Mercier, L. (1994a) Validation of the Box and Block test as a measure of dexterity of elderly people: Reliability, validity, and norms studies. Archives of Physical Medicine and Rehabilitation; 75:751-755

Desrosiers, J., Hébert, R., Bravo, G., Dutil, E. (1995a) Upper Extremity Performance Test for the Elderly (TEMPA): Normative data and correlates with sensorimotor parameters. Archives of Physical Medicine and Rehabilitation; 76:1125-1129

Desrosiers, J., Hébert, R., Bravo, G., Dutil, E. (1995b) The Purdue Pegboard Test: Normative data for people aged 60 and over. Disability and Rehabilitation; 17:217-24

Desrosiers, J., Hébert, R., Dutil, E., Bravo, G. (1993) Development and reliability of an upper extremity function test for the elderly: The TEMPA. Canadian Journal of Occupational Therapy; 60:9-16

Desrosiers, J., Hébert, R., Dutil, E., Bravo, G., Mercier, L. (1994b) Validity of the TEMPA: A measurement instrument for upper extremity performance. Occupational Journal of Research; 14:267-281

Desrosiers, J., Rochette, A., Hebert, R., Bravo, G. (1997) The Minnesota Manual Dexterity: Reliability, validity and reference values studies with healthy elderly people. Canadian Journal of Occupational Therapy; 64:270-276

Deyo, R.A., Diehr, P., Patrick, D.L. (1991) Reproducibility and responsiveness of health status measures. Statistics and strategies for evaluation. Control Clin Trials; 12:142-158

Dickerson, A.E., Fisher, A.G. (1993) Age differences in functional performance. Am J Occup Ther, 47:686-92

Dickerson, A.E., Fisher, A.G. (1995) Culture-relevant functional performance assessment of Hispanic elderly. Occup Ther J Res, 15:50-68

Doble, S.E., Fisk, J.D., Fisher, A.G., Ritvo, P.G., Murray, T.J. (1994) Evaluation functional competence of community-dwelling persons with multiple sclerosis using the Assessment of Motor and Process Skills (AMPS). Arch Phys Med Rehabil; 75:843-51

Duncan, P.W., Goldstein, L.B., Matchar, D., Divine, G., Feussner J. (1992) Measurement of motor recovery after stroke. Outcome assessment and sample size requirements. Stroke; 23:1084-9

Duncan, P.W., Propst, M., Nelson, S.G. (1983) Reliability of the Fugl-Meyer assessment of sensorimotor recovery following cerebrovascular accident. Phys Ther; 63:1607-1610

Dutil, E., Filiatrault, J, De Serres, L., Arsenault, A.B. (1990) Evaluation de la fonction du membre supérieur chez le sujet hémiplegique – Protocol d'évaluation [Evaluation of upper extremity function in subjects with hemiplegia]. Montreal: Librairie de l'Université de Montréal

Emerson, S. (1993) Validity of the Jebsen Hand Function Test. J Hand Ther; 6:65-66

Epstein, A.A. (1995) The outcome movement: will it get us where we want to go? In: Graham, N.O. (ed.), Quality in health care. Theory, application, and evolution. Gaithersburg: Aspen Publishers, pp. 188-197.

Feys, H., De Weerdt, W., Nuyens, G., Van de Winckel, A., Selz, B., Kiekens, C. (2000) Predicting motor recovery of the upper limb after stroke rehabilitation: value of a clinical examination. Physiotherapy Research International; 5:1-18

Filiatrault, J., Arsenault, A.B., Dutil, E., D. Bourbonnais (1991) Motor function and activities of daily living assessments: A study of three tests for persons with hemiplegia. American Journal of Occupational Therapy; 45:806-810

Fisher A. Assessment of Motor and Process Skills Manual (research ed. 7.0) (unpublished test manual). Fort Collins, CO: Colorado State University 1994

Fisher, A.G. (1993) The Assessment of IADL motor skills: An application of many-faceted Rasch analysis. Am J Occup Ther; 47:319-29

Fisher, A.G. (1994b) Development of a functional assessment that adjusts ability measures for task simplicity and rater leniency. In: Wilson, M., editor. Objective measurement. Theory and practice, vol. 2. Norwood, NJ: Ablex, 145-175

Fisher, A.G. (1995) Assessment of Motor and Process Skills. Ft. Collins, CO: Three Star Press

Fisher, A.G., Lui, Y., Velozo, C.A., Pan, A.W. (1992) Cross-cultural assessment of process skills. Am J Occup Ther; 46:876-85

Fitts, P.M. (1954) The information capacity of the human motor system in controlling the amplitude of movement. J Exp Psychol; 47:381-391

Fraser, C., Defusco, J. (1981) A standardized test of hand function. Br J Occup Ther; 44:258-260

Fugl-Meyer, A.R. (1976a) Assessment of motor function in hemiplegic patients. In: Buerger, A.A. (ed): Neurophysiologic aspects of Rehabilitation Medicine. Charles C. Thomas, Springfield, IL, chapter 15

Fugl-Meyer, A.R. (1976b) The effect of rehabilitation in hemiplegia as reflected in the relation between motor recovery and ADL function. Proceedings International Rehabilitation Association II, Mexico City, 683

Fugl-Meyer, A.R. (1980) Post-stroke hemiplegia: Assessment of physical properties. Scand J Rehabil Med; Suppl 7:85-93

Fugl-Meyer, A.R., Jääskö, L. (1980) Post-stroke hemiplegia and ADL-performance. Scand J Rehab Med; Suppl 7:140-152

Fugl-Meyer, A.R., Jääskö, L., Leyman, I., Olsson, S., Steglind, S. (1975) The post-stroke hemiplegic patient. Scand J Rehab Med; 7:13-31

Fugl-Meyer, A.R., Steger, H.G., Jääskö, L., Loid, M. (1976c) Return to work with hemiplegia. Proc. IRMA II (Mexico City, 1974):703

Goodkin, D., Priore, R., Wende, K. (1998) Comparing the ability of various composive outcomes to discriminate treatment effects in MS clinical trials. The multiple sclerosis Collaborative Research Group (MSCRG). Multiple Sclerosis, 4:480-6

Goodkin, D.E., Hertsgaard, D., Seminary, J. (1988) Upper extremity function in Multiple Sclerosis: Improving assessment sensitivity with Box-and-Block and Nine-Hole Peg Tests. Arch Phys Med Rehabil; 69:850-854

Haaland, K.Y., Delaney, H.D. (1981) Motor deficit after left or right hemisphere damage due to stroke or tumor. Neuropsychologia; 19:17-27

Hackel, M.E., Wolfe, G.A., Bang, S.M., Canfield, J.S. (1992) Changes in hand function in the ageing adult as determined by the Jebsen Test of Hand Function. Phys Ther; 72:373-377

Hamm, N.H., Curtis, D. (1980) Normative data for the Purdue Pegboard on a sample of adult candidates for vocational rehabilitation. Perceptual and Motor Skills; 50:309-310

Hantson, L., de Weerdt, W., de Kayser, J., Diener, H.C., Franke, C., Palm, R., Van Orshoven, M., Schoonderwalt, H., de Klippel, N., Herroelen, L., Feys, H. (1994) The European stroke scale. Stroke; 25:2215-2219

Hébert, R., Carrier, R., Bilodeau, A. (1988) The functional autonomy measurement system (SMAF): Description and validation of an instrument for the measurement of handicaps. Age and Ageing; 17:293-302

Heller, A., Wade, D.T., Wood, V.A., Sunderland, A., Hewer, R.L., Ward, E. (1987) Arm function after stroke: Measurement and recovery over the first three months. Journal of Neurology, Neurosurgery, and Psychiatry; 50:714-719

Hicks, C.M.: Research methods for clinical therapists. Applied project design and analysis. Churchill Livingstone, Edinburgh, 1999, 3rd edition

Hines, M., O'Connor, J. (1926) A measure of finger dexterity. Personnel J; 4:379-382

Hsieh, C.-L., Hsueh, I.-P., Chiang, F.-M., Lin, P.-H. (1998) Interrater reliability and validity of the Action Research Arm test in stroke patients. Age-Ageing; 27:107-114

Hsueh, I.P., Hsieh, C.L. (2002) Responsiveness of two upper extremity function instruments for stroke inpatients receiving rehabilitation. Clin Rehabil; 16:617-624

Hsueh, I.P., Lee, M.M., Hsieh, C.L. (2001) Psychometric characteristics of the Barthel activities of daily living index in stroke patients. J Formos Med Assoc; 100:526-532

Instructions and Normative Data for Model 32020 Purdue Pegboard. Lafayette Instrument Company

Jebsen, R.H., Taylor, N., Trieschmann, R.B., Trotter, M.J., Howard, L.A. (1969) An objective and standardized test of hand function. Arch Phys Med Rehabil; 50:311-349

Jones, R.D., Donaldson, I.M., Parkin, P.J. (1989) Impairment and recovery of ipsilateral sensory-motor function following unilateral cerebral infarction. Brain, 12:113-32

Kaegi, C., Thibault, M.-C., Giroux, F., Bourbonnais, D. (1998) The interrater reliability of force measurements using a modified sphygmomanometer in elderly subjects. Physical Therapy; 78:1095-1103

Kellor, M., Frost, J., Silberberg, N., Iversen, I., Cummings, R. (1971) Hand strength and dexterity. American Journal of Occupational Therapy, 25:77-83

Kopp, B., Kunkel, A., Flor, H., Platz, T., Rose, U., Mauritz, K.-H., Gresser, K., McCulloch, K.L., Taub E. (1997) The Arm Motor Ability Test (AMAT): Reliability, validity and sensitivity to change of an instrument for assessing disabilities in the activities of daily living. Archives of Physical Medicine and Rehabilitation; 78:615-620

Kurtzke, J.F. (1970) Neurologic impairment in Multiple Sclerosis and the Disability Status Scale. Acta Neurol Scand; 46:493-512

Kurtzke, J.F. (1983) Rating neurologic impairment in multiple sclerosis: An expanded disability status scale (EDDS). Neurology; 33:1444-1452

Kusoffsky, H., Wadell, I., Nilsson, B.Y. (1982) The relationship between sensory impairment and motor recovery in patients with hemiplegia. Scandinavian Journal of Rehabilitation Medicine; 14:27-32

Langhammer, B. and Stanghelle, J.K. (2000) Bobath or Motor Relearning Programme ? A comparison of two different approaches of physiotherapy in stroke rehabilitation: a randomized controlled study. Clinical Rehabilitation; 14:361-369.

Levin, H.S., High, W.M., Goethe, K.E., Sisson, R.A., Overall, J.E., Rhoades, H.M., Eisenberg, R.M., Kalisky, Z., Gary, H.E. (1987) The neurobehavioral rating scale: assessment of the behavioral sequelae fo head injury by the clinician. J Neurol Neurosurg Psychiatry; 50:183-193

Lin, F.-M., Sabbahi, M. (1999) Correlation of spasticity with hyperactive stretch reflexes and motor dysfunction in hemiplegia. Arch Phys Med Rehabil; 80:526-530

Lin, J.H., Hsueh, I.P., Sheu, C.F., Hsieh, C.L. (2004) Psychometric properties of the sensory scale of the Fugl-Meyer Assessment in stroke patients. Clin Rehabil, 18:391-397

Lincoln, N., Leadbitter, D. (1979) Assessment of motor function in stroke patients. Physiotherapy, 65:48-51

Lindmark, B., Hamrin, E. (1988) Evaluation of functional capacity after stroke as a basis for active intervention. Scand J Rehabil Med; 20:111-115

Loewen, S.C., Anderson, B.A (1990) Predictors of stroke outcome using objective measurement scales. Stroke; 21:78-81

Loewen, S.C., Anderson, B.A. (1988) Reliability of modified motor assessment scale and the Barthel Index. Phys Ther, 68:1077-1081

Lyle, R.C. (1981) A performance test for assessment of upper limb function in physical rehabilitation treatment and research. Int J Rehab Research; 4:483-492

Malouin, F., Pichard, L., Bonneau, C., Durand, A., Corriveau, D. (1994) Evaluating motor recovery early after stroke: Comparison of the Fugl-Meyer Assessment and the Motor Assessment Scale. Arch Phys Med Rehabil; 75:1206-1212

Marque, Ph., Felez, A., Puel, M., Demonet, J.F., Guiraud-Chaumeil, B., Roques, C.F., Chollet, F. (1997) Impairment and recovery of left motor function in patients with right hemiplegia. Journal of Neurology, Neurosurgery, and Psychiatry; 62:77-81

Masur, H. Skalen und Scores in der Neurologie. Stuttgart, New York, Thieme Verlag 2000, 2. Aufl., german

Mathiowetz, V., Kashman, N., Volland, G., Weber, K., Dowe, M., Rogers, S. (1985a) Grip and pinch strength: Normative data for adults. Archives of Phys Med Rehabil; 66:69-72

Mathiowetz, V., Volland, G., Kashman, N., Weber, K. (1985c) Adult Norms for the Box and Block Test of manual dexterity. American Journal of Occupational Therapy; 39:386-391

Mathiowetz, V., Weber, K., Kashman, N., Volland, G. (1985b) Adult norms for Nine Hole Peg Test of finger dexterity. Occup Ther J Res; 5:25-38

McCulloch, K., Cook, E.W., Fleming, W.C., Novack, T.A., Nepomuceno, C.S., Taub, E. (1988) A reliable test of upper extremity ADL function (abstract). Archives of Physical Medicine and Rehabilitation; 69:755

Miltner, W.H.R., Bauder, H., Sommer, M., Dettmers, C., and Taub, E. (1999) Effects of constraint-induced movement therapy on patients with chronic motor deficits after stroke. A replication. Stroke; 30: 586-92.

Nelles, G., Jentzen, W., Jueptner, M., Müller, S., and Diener, H.C. (2001) Arm training induced brain plasticity in stroke studied wih serial positron emission tomography. NeuroImage; 13: 1146-1154.

Nygard, L., Bernspang, B., Fisher, A.G., Winblad, B. (1994) Comparing motor and process ability of persons with suspected dementia in home and clinic settings. American Journal of Occupational Therapy; 48:689-696

O`Connor, D., Kortman, B., Smith, A., Ahern, M., Smith, M., Krishnan, J. (1999) Correlation between objective and subjective measures of hand function in patient with rheumatoid arthritis. J Hand Ther, 12:323-329

Oldfield, R.C. (1971) The assessment and analysis of handedness: The Edinburgh Inventory. Neuropsychologia; 9:97-113

Park, S., Fisher, A.G., Velozo, C.A. (1994) Using the assessment of motor and process skills to compare occupational performance between clinic and home settings. Am J Occup Ther, 48:697-709

Parker, V.M., Wade, D.T., Langton-Hewer, R. (1986) Loss of arm function after stroke: measurement, frequency, and recovery. International Rehabilitation Medicine; 8:69-73

Platz, T., Prass, K., Denzler, P., Bock, S., Mauritz, K.-H. (1999) Testing a motor performance series and a kinematic motion analysis as measures of performance in high functioning stroke patients: reliability, validity, and responsiveness to therapeutic intervention. Arch Phys Med Rehabil; 80:270-277

Platz, T., Winter, T., Müller, N., Pinkowski, C., Eickhof, C., Mauritz, K.-H. (2001) Arm Ability Training for Stroke and Traumatic Brain Injury Patients with mild arm paresis. A Single-Blind, Randomized, Controlled Trial. Archives of Physical Medicine and Rehabilitation; 82: 961-968.

Platz, T., Denzler, P. (2002) Do psychological variables modify motor recovery among patients with mild arm paresis after stroke or traumatic brain injury who receive the Arm Ability training ? Restorative Neurology and Neuroscience; 20: 37-49.

Platz, T., Kim, I.-H., Engel, U., Kieselbach, A., and Mauritz, K.-H. (2002) Brain activation pattern as assessed with multi-modal EEG analysis predict motor recovery among stroke patients with mild arm paresis who receive the Arm Ability training. Restorative Neurology and Neuroscience; 20: 21-35.

Platz, T., Pinkowski, C., van Wijck, F., Kim, I.-H., di Bella, P., Johnson, G. (2005) Reliability and validity of arm function assessment with standardised guidelines for the Fugl-Meyer Test, Action Research Arm Test and Box and Block Test: a multi-centre study. Clinical Rehabil; 19:404-411.

Platz, T., Eickhof, C., van Kaick, S., Engel, U., Pinkowski, C., Kalok, S., and Pause, M. Impairment-oriented training or Bobath therapy for arm paresis after stroke: a single blind, multi-centre randomized controlled trial. Clin Rehabil, in press [a].

Platz, T., van Kaick, S., Möller, L., Freund, S., Winter, T., and Kim, I.-H. Impairment-oriented training and adaptive motor cortex reorganisation after stroke: a fTMS study. J Neurol, in press [b]

Poole, J.L., Whitney, S.L. (1988) Motor Assessment Scale for stroke patients: concurrent validity and interrater reliability. Arch Phys Med Rehabil; 69:195-197

Provinciali, L., Ceravolo, M.G., Bartolini, M., Logullo, F., Danni, M. (1999) A multidimensional assessment of multiple sclerosis: relationships between disability domains. Acta Neurol Scand; 100:156-162

Rapin, L., Tourk, L.M., Costa, L.D. (1966) Evaluation of the Purdue Pegboard as a screening test for brain damage. Developmental Medicine and Child Neurology; 8:45-54

Reynolds, G., Archibald, K.C., Brunnström, S, Thompson, N. (1958) Preliminary report on neuromuscular function testing of the upper extremity in adult hemiplegic patients. Arch Phys Med; 39:303

Roberts, L., Counsell, C. (1998) Assessment of clinical outcomes in acute stroke trials. Stroke; 29:986-991

Rödén-Jüllig, A., Gustafsson, C., Fugl-Meyer, A. (1994) Validation of four scales for the acute stage of stroke. J Internal Med; 236:125-136

Rosen, B., Dahlin, L.B., Lundborg, G. (2000) Assessment of functional outcome after nerve repair in a longitudinal cohort. Scand J Plast Reconstr Surg Hand Surg; 34:71-78

Rudman, D., Hannah, S. (1998) An instrument evaluation framework: Description and application to assessments of hand function. Journal of Hand Therapy; 11:266-277

Sanford, J., Moreland, J., Swanson, L.R., Stratford, P.W., Gowland, C. (1993) Reliability of the Fugl-Meyer Assessment for testing motor performance in patients following stroke. Physical Therapy; 73:447-454

Schoppe, K.-J. (1974) Das MLS-Gerät: Ein neuer Testapparat zur Messung feinmotorischer Leistungen. Sonderdruck aus Diagnostica XX/1:43-46, german

Sharpless, J.W. The nine-hole peg test of finger hand co-ordination for the hemiplegic patient. In: Sharpless J.W., ed. Mossman's A Problem Oriented Approach to Stroke Rehabilitation. Springfield, Illinois: Charles C. Thomas; 1982:420-423

Siegel, M., Hirschorn, B. (1958) Adolescent norms for the Purdue Pegboard Tests. Personnel and Guidance Journal; 36:363-365

Sjögren, K., Fugl-Meyer, A.R. (1982) Adjustment to life after stroke. With special reference to sexual intercourse and leisure. J Psychosom Res; 26:409

Smith, H.B. (1973) Smith Hand Function Evaluation. Am J Occup Ther, 27; 244-251

Sollerman, C., Ejeskar, A. (1995) Sollerman hand function test. A standardised method and its use in tetraplegic patients. Scand J Plast Reconstr Surg Hand Surg; 29:167-176

Spaulding, S.J., McPhearson, J.J., Strachota, E.S., Kuphal, M., Ramponi, M. (1988) Jebsen Hand Function Test: Performance of the uninvolved hand in hemiplegia and of right-handed, right and left hemiplegic persons. Arch Phys Med Rehabil; 69:419-422

Spreen, O., Strauss, E.E. A compendium of neuropsychological tests: administration, norms and commentary. London: Oxford Medicine, 1991

Sturm, W., Büssing, A. (1985) Ergänzende Normierungsdaten und Retest-Reliabilitätskoeffizienten zur motorischen Leistungsserie (MLS) nach Schoppe. Diagnostica; 3:234-245

Sunderland, A., Tinson, D., Bradley, L., Hewer, R.L. (1989) Arm function after stroke. An evaluation of grip strength as a measure of recovery and a prognostic indicator. Journal of Neurology, Neurosurgery and Psychiatry; 52:1267-72

Sunderland, A., Tinson, D.J., Bradley, E.L., Fletcher, D. Langton Hewer, R., Wade, D.T. (1992) Enhanced physical therapy improves recovery of arm function after stroke. A randomised controlled trial. Journal of Neurology, Neurosurgery, and Psychiatry; 55:530-535

Teasdale, G., Jennet, B. (1974) Assessment of coma and impaired consciousness. A practical scale. Lancet; (ii):81-83

Tiffin, J. (1948) Purdue Pegboard Examiner Manual. Chicago, IL: Science Research Associates

Tiffin, J., Asher, E.J. (1948) The Purdue Pegboard: Norms and studies of reliability and validity. Journal of Applied Psychology; 32:234-47

Turton, A.J., Fraser, C.M. (1986) A test battery to measure the recovery of voluntary movement control following stroke. Int Rehabil Med; 8:74-78

Twitchell, T.E. (1951) The restoration of motor function following hemiplegia in man. Brain; 74:443

van Buskirk, C. (1954) Return of motor function in hemiplegia. Neurology; 4:919-928

van der Lee, J.H., Beckermann, H., Lankhorst, G.J., Bouter, L.M. (2001) The responsiveness of the Action Research Arm test and the Fugl-Meyer Assessment scale in chronic stroke patients. J Rehabil Med; 33:110-113

van der Lee, J.H., de Groot, V., Beckermann, H., Wagenaar, R.C., Lankhorst, G.J., and Bouter, L.M. (2001) The intra- and interrater reliability of the Action Research Arm test: a practical test of upper extremity function in patients with stroke. Arch Phys Med Rehabil; 82: 14-19.

van der Lee, J.H., Beckermann, H., Knol, D.L., de Vet, H.C., Bouter, L.M. (2004) Clinimetric properties of the motor activity log for the assessment of arm use in hemiparetic patients. Stroke 35:1410-1414

van Wijck, F., Pandyan, A.D., Johnson, G.R., Barnes, M.P. (2001) Assessing motor deficits in neurological rehabilitation: patterns of instrument usage. Neurorehabilitation and Neural Repair; 15:23-30.

Vega, A. (1969) Use of Purdue pegboard and finger tapping performance as a rapid screening test for brain damage. J Clin Physiol; 25:255-8

Wade, D.T., Langton Hewer, R. (1987) Motor loss and swallowing difficulty after stroke: frequency, recovery and prognosis. Acta Neurol Scand; 76:50-54

Wade, D.T.: Measurement in neurological rehabilitation. Oxford University Press, Oxford, New York, Tokyo, 1992

Wade, D.T., Langton Hewer, R., Wood, V.A., Skilbeck, C.E., Ismail, H.M. (1983) The hemiplegic arm after stroke: measurement and recovery. J Neurol Neurosurg Psychiatrie; 46:521-524

Walker-Batson, D.W., Smith, P., Curtis, S., Unwin, H., Greenlee, R. (1995) Amphetamine paired with physical therapy accelerates motor recovery after stroke. Stroke; 26: 2254-2259.

Wang, C.H., Hsieh, C.L., Dai, M.H., Chen, C.H., Lai, Y.F. Inter-rater reliability and validity of the stroke rehabilitation assessment of movement (stream) instrument. J Rehabil Med; 34:20-24

Whetsell, G.W. (1995) Total quality management. In: Graham NO (ed.), Quality in health care. Theory, application, and evolution. Gaithersburg: Aspen Publishers, 1995, pp. 79-91.

WHO (2001). The ICF (International Classification of Functioning, Disability and Health). Geneva: World Health Organization.

Wilson, D.J., Baker, L.L., Craddock, J.A. (1984a) Functional test for the hemiparetic upper extremity. American Journal of Occupational Therapy; 38:159-164

Wilson, D.J., Baker, L.L., Craddock, J.A. (1984b) Protocol-Functional Test for the Hemiplegic/Paretic Upper Extremity. Downey, C.A.: Rancho Los Amigos Occupational Therapy Department and Rehabilitation Engineering Centre

Wood-Dauphinee, S., Williams, J.I., Shapiro, S.H. (1990) Examining outcome measures in a clinical study of stroke. Stroke; 21:731-739

Yelnik, A., Bonan, I., Debray, M., Lo, E., Gelbert, F., Bussel, B. (1996) Changes in the execution of a complex manual task after ipsilateral ischemic cerebral hemispheric stroke. Archives of Physical Medicine and Rehabilitation; 77:806-10

# 7. Acknowledgements

The authors are indebted to staff of the clinical centres that contributed to the reliability and validity study, from the Charité – Universitätsmedizin Berlin, Department of Neurological Rehabilitation, Germany; from Hunters Moor Regional Neurological Rehabilitation, Department of Neurorehabilitation at the University of Newcastle upon Tyne, U.K.; from the Centro per lo Studio ed il Trattamento dei Neurolesi Lungodegenti, Messina, Italy; from the Rehabilitation Department, National Multiple Sclerosis Centre, Melsbroek, Belgium. Individuals are named in the original publication (Platz et al., 2005). Peter Feys, P.T., from the National Multiple Sclerosis Centre, Melsbroek, Belgium, helped also with the design of score sheets.

The authors are further indebted to C. Eickhof, P.T., S. Freund, M.D., and S. van Kaick, P.T., M.Sc., for their demonstration of test items on photos.

This book was developed under the EU funded program: DE4203, DRAMA - Developments in Rehabilitation of the Arm – within the TELEMATICS APPLICATIONS PROGRAMME (Disabled and Elderly). Manuscript preparation was supported by a grant from the German Federal Minister for Education and Research to TP within the framework of the competence net 'stroke'.

# 8. Score sheets, electronic data base with electronic score sheets, and demonstration videos

Score sheets for the FM, ARAT and the BBT are presented next. Please contact the first author (e.g. web site http://userpage.fu-berlin.de/~tplatz/) for further information regarding electronic FM score sheets embedded in an electronic database and for demonstration videos (on CD or DVD) for the FM, ARAT, and the BBT.

## FUGL-MEYER ARM SCORE

Patient:            Centre:

Examiner:        Date :

Assessed side: left ☐ or right ☐

| A. SHOULDER-ELBOW-FOREARM<br>(patient sitting) | | |
|---|---|---|
| **I REFLEX-ACTIVITY**<br><br>*Biceps, Triceps, Fingerflexors* | - no reflex-activity         ☐ 0<br>- reflex-activity in biceps and/or<br>  fingerflexors            ☐ 2<br><br>- no reflex-activity         ☐ 0<br>- reflex-activity in extensors   ☐ 2 | **/4** |
| **II VOLITIONAL MOVEMENTS WITHIN DYNAMIC SYNERGIES**<br>(patient sitting with the back against the backrest)<br><br>*a) Flexor synergy:* "hand to your (ipsilateral) ear" with shoulder retraction<br>                forearm<br>                elbow<br>                shoulder<br><br>*b) Extensor synergy:* "knuckles on contralateral knee" from flexor synergy (with support, if needed)<br>Make sure that the knees are placed apart.<br>                forearm<br>                elbow<br>                shoulder |                   none   partial  perfect<br>supination:      ☐ 0    ☐ 1    ☐ 2<br>flexion:          ☐ 0    ☐ 1    ☐ 2<br>outw rotation:   ☐ 0    ☐ 1    ☐ 2<br>abduction (90°):  ☐ 0    ☐ 1    ☐ 2<br>elevation:      ☐ 0    ☐ 1    ☐ 2<br>retraction:     ☐ 0    ☐ 1    ☐ 2<br><br><br>pronation:      ☐ 0    ☐ 1    ☐ 2<br>extension:     ☐ 0    ☐ 1    ☐ 2<br>adduction + int rotation ☐ 0  ☐ 1  ☐ 2 | **/18** |
| **III VOLITIONAL MOVEMENTS WITHIN A MIX OF DYNAMIC SYNERGIES**<br>*a) Hand to lumbar spine*<br>"bring your hand on your back" Patient seated towards the front of the chair. | - hand not behind spina iliaca ant. sup.  ☐ 0<br>- hand behind spina iliaca ant. sup., without<br>  any gravitational tricks         ☐ 1<br>- perfect                         ☐ 2 | |
| *b) Shoulder flexion 0° to 90°*<br>elbow extended, forearm in midposition<br>"bring your extended arm up, thumb upwards". The examiner may assist the patient to get into the starting position. | - arm immediately in abduction or elbow in<br>  flexion                        ☐ 0<br>- arm not immediately in abduction and/or<br>  elbow in flexion              ☐ 1<br>- perfect                         ☐ 2 | |
| *c) Pro-Supination of the forearm*<br>elbow flexed 90°, shoulder 0°<br>The patient has to reach this position without support. Score against passive RoM.<br>Beware of any compensation in the glenohumeral joint. | - starting position impossible and/or no pro-<br>  supination                    ☐ 0<br>- starting position possible and kept during the<br>  movement, limited pro-supination  ☐ 1<br>- perfect                       ☐ 2 | **/6** |

*From:* ARM Arm Rehabilitation Measurement, © Thomas Platz, 2005

| | | |
|---|---|---|
| **IV VOLITIONAL MOVEMENTS WITH LITTLE OR NO SYNERGY DEPENDENCE**<br><br>*a) Shoulder abduction 0 - 90°*<br>elbow fully extended and forearm pronated<br>The examiner may assist the patient to get into the starting position. | - arm immediately supinated and/or elbow flexed ☐0<br><br>- motion only partly or elbow is flexed or the forearm can not be kept in the pronated position ☐ 1<br>- perfect ☐ 2 | |
| *b) Shoulder flexion 90° to 180°*<br>arm in 0° abduction, elbow extended and forearm in midposition, "bring extended arm up, thumb up"<br>The examiner may assist the patient to get into the starting position. | - arm immediately in abd. or elbow flexed ☐ 0<br>- arm not immediately in abduction and/or elbow in flexion ☐ 1<br>- perfect ☐ 2 | |
| *c) Pro-Supination of the forearm*<br>shoulder 30° - 90° flexion, elbow in extension<br>The patient has to reach this position without support. Score against passive RoM.<br>Beware of any compensation in the glenohumeral joint. | - starting position impossible and/or no pro-sup ☐ 0<br>- starting position possible and kept during the movement, limited pro-sup ☐ 1<br>- perfect ☐ 2 | **/6** |
| **V NORMAL REFLEX-ACTIVITIES**<br>Only assessed if in the previous section total score = 6 | a) not assessed (because score of A. IV < 6) ☐ 0<br>b) assessed:<br>- = 2 of 3 reflex-activities are markedly hyperactive ☐ 0<br>- 1 reflex markedly hyperactive or = 2 lively ☐ 1<br>- no hyperactive reflexes ☐ 2 | **/2** |
| **B. WRIST**<br>The patient seated has to perform the wrist items partly with the elbow flexed to 90° and partly with the elbow fully extended,. the shoulder should be in 0° position. The examiner may assist the patient to get and keep these positions. | | |
| *a) Wrist stability in 15° dorsal flexion*<br>shoulder 0°, elbow 90°, forearm fully pronated | - dorsiflexion to required position not possible ☐ 0<br>- required position possible, no resistance ☐ 1<br>- required position can be maintained against some (slight) resistance ☐ 2 | |
| *b) Repeated wrist flexion - extension*<br>shoulder in 0°, elbow 90°, forearm pronated<br>Score against passive RoM. | - no active repeated movements ☐ 0<br>- active movements smaller than passive movements ☐ 1<br>- detail is fully and adequately performed ☐ 2 | |
| *c) Wrist stability in 15° dorsiflexion*<br>shoulder slightly flexed and/or abducted, elbow extended, forearm pronated. | - dorsiflexion to required position not possible ☐ 0<br>- required wrist position possible, no resistance ☐ 1<br>- required position can be maintained against some (slight) resistance ☐ 2 | |
| *d) Repeated wrist flexion - extension*<br>shoulder slightly flexed and/or abducted, elbow extended, forearm pronated.<br>Score against passive RoM. | - no active repeated movements ☐ 0<br>- active movements smaller than passive movements ☐ 1<br>- detail is fully and adequately performed ☐ 2 | |
| *e) Circumduction of the wrist*<br>shoulder 0°, elbow 90°. Examiner may provide support for the forearm but not restrain it. | - impossible ☐ 0<br>- jerky or incomplete movements ☐ 1<br>- detail is fully and adequately performed ☐ 2 | **/10** |

From: ARM Arm Rehabilitation Measurement, © Thomas Platz, 2005

## C. HAND

Seven details are evaluated. Of these, five are grasps with different types of muscular co-contractions. This section of the Fugl-Meyer focuses on the ability of the patient to perform <u>active movements</u>. The examiner may, if necessary, support the elbow of the seated patient in the 90° position; no support may be given for the wrist.

| <u>a) Flexion of the fingers</u> | - no flexion ☐ 0<br>- some, but not full active flexion ☐ 1<br>- full active flexion compared with the<br>  unaffected hand ☐ 2 |
|---|---|
| <u>b) Extension of the fingers</u><br>from the position of full flexion (eventually passive) | - no extension ☐ 0<br>- some, but not full ext. or release of an active<br>  mass flexion grasp ☐ 1<br>- full active extension, compared with the<br>  unaffected hand ☐ 2 |

### Grasp tests:

All grasp tests consist of an active (i.e. grasping) and static (i.e. holding against resistance) component which can be clearly distinguished, the required position should be maintained during the tug.

| <u>c) Grasp A: extension MCP, flexion PIP and DIP</u><br>grasp has to be maintained against resistance | - required position not possible ☐ 0<br>- weak grasp ☐ 1<br>- grasp maintained against relatively great<br>  resistance ☐ 2 |
|---|---|
| <u>d) Grasp B: extended index and thumb</u><br>(holding a sheet with the volar side of the extended thumb and the metacarpale of the index finger against a horizontal tug away from the patient) | - the function as such can not be performed ☐ 0<br>- scrap of paper kept in place, not against a<br>  slight tug ☐ 1<br>- scrap of paper is held well against a tug ☐ 2 |
| <u>e) Grasp C: pulpa of the thumb against the pulpa of the index</u><br>(holding a pencil with the pulpae of thumb and index finger against an upwards tug) | - the function as such can not be performed ☐ 0<br>- pencil kept in place, not against a slight tug ☐ 1<br>- pencil is held well against a tug ☐ 2 |
| <u>f) Grasp D: volar surface of the thumb and index against each other</u><br>(holding a cylinder-shaped object against an upwards tug) | - the function as such can not be performed ☐ 0<br>- cylinder kept in place, not against a slight tug ☐ 1<br>- cylinder is held well against a tug ☐ 2 |
| <u>g) Grasp E: spherical grasp</u><br>(grasping a tennisball and holding it against a downwards tug) | - the function as such can not be performed ☐ 0<br>- ball grasped, not held against a slight tug ☐ 1<br>- ball grasped, well held against a tug ☐ 2 |

/14

*From:* ARM Arm Rehabilitation Measurement, © Thomas Platz, 2005

| D. CO-ORDINATION/ SPEED | | | | |
|---|---|---|---|---|
| **Finger-to-nose test:**<br>Starting position with the elbow fully extended and the shoulder in 90° abduction | | | | |
| a) T*remor* | marked<br>☐ 0 | slight<br>☐ 1 | no<br>☐ 2 | |
| b) *Dysmetria* | pronounced or unsystematic<br>☐ 0 | slight and systematic<br>☐ 1 | no<br>☐ 2 | |
| c) *Time*<br>    compare time affected to unaffected side | > 6 sec<br>☐ 0<br><br>time right:<br>                    sec. | 2-5 sec<br>☐ 1<br><br>time left:<br>                    sec. | < 2 sec<br>☐ 2 | /6 |
| | **TOTAL MOTOR FUNCTION;<br>UPPER LIMB** | | | /66 |

| H. SENSATION | | | | |
|---|---|---|---|---|
| **a) Light touch**<br>Ask the patient whether she/he feels that light touch on both arms and the palmar surface of the hands gave the same qualitative and quantitative impression.<br><br>Score light touch as follows:<br>0:      anaesthesia<br>1:      hypaesthesia, dysaesthesia<br>2:      normaesthesia<br><br>- volar side of the forearm<br>- palmar surface of the hand | <br><br><br><br><br><br><br><br><br>☐ 0<br>☐ 0 | <br><br><br><br><br><br><br><br><br>☐ 1<br>☐ 1 | <br><br><br><br><br><br><br><br><br>☐ 2<br>☐ 2 | |

| _b) Position sense of the joints_ | | | | |
|---|---|---|---|---|
| Patient blindfolded. Score position sense of the joints as follows:<br>0:   absence of sensation<br>1:   considerable difference compared with the<br>     joint on the unaffected side, but at least ¾<br>     of the answers correct<br>2:   all answers correct, little or no difference<br>     comparing unaffected with affected limb | | | | |
| - glenohumeral joint | ☐ 0 | ☐ 1 | ☐ 2 | |
| - elbow | ☐ 0 | ☐ 1 | ☐ 2 | |
| - wrist | ☐ 0 | ☐ 1 | ☐ 2 | |
| - thumb (interphalangeal joint) | ☐ 0 | ☐ 1 | ☐ 2 | |
| **TOTAL SENSATION, UPPER LIMB** | | | | **/12** |

| _J. PASSIVE JOINT MOTION/JOINT PAIN_ | | | | | |
|---|---|---|---|---|---|
| _a) Passive joint motion_ | | | | | |
| Score passive joint motion as follows:<br>0:   only few degrees of range-of-motion<br>1:   decreased passive range-of-motion<br>2:   normal passive range-of-motion | | | | | |
| Shoulder | flexion | ☐ 0 | ☐ 1 | ☐ 2 | |
| | abduction to 90 ° | ☐ 0 | ☐ 1 | ☐ 2 | |
| | outw. rotation | ☐ 0 | ☐ 1 | ☐ 2 | |
| | inw. rotation | ☐ 0 | ☐ 1 | ☐ 2 | |
| Elbow | flexion | ☐ 0 | ☐ 1 | ☐ 2 | |
| | extension | ☐ 0 | ☐ 1 | ☐ 2 | |
| Forearm | pronation | ☐ 0 | ☐ 1 | ☐ 2 | |
| | supination | ☐ 0 | ☐ 1 | ☐ 2 | |
| Wrist | flexion | ☐ 0 | ☐ 1 | ☐ 2 | |
| | extension | ☐ 0 | ☐ 1 | ☐ 2 | |
| Fingers | flexion | ☐ 0 | ☐ 1 | ☐ 2 | **/24** |
| | extension | ☐ 0 | ☐ 1 | ☐ 2 | |

| | | | | | |
|---|---|---|---|---|---|
| **b) Joint pain** <br> Score occurrence of joint pain as follows: <br> 0:    pronounced pain during all the movement <br>      or very marked pain at the end of the <br>      actual range of motion <br> 1:    some pain <br> 2:    no pain | | | | | |
| Shoulder | flexion <br> abduction to 90 ° <br> outw. rotation <br> inw. rotation | ☐ 0 <br> ☐ 0 <br> ☐ 0 <br> ☐ 0 | ☐ 1 <br> ☐ 1 <br> ☐ 1 <br> ☐ 1 | ☐ 2 <br> ☐ 2 <br> ☐ 2 <br> ☐ 2 | |
| Elbow | flexion <br> extension | ☐ 0 <br> ☐ 0 | ☐ 1 <br> ☐ 1 | ☐ 2 <br> ☐ 2 | |
| Forearm | pronation <br> supination | ☐ 0 <br> ☐ 0 | ☐ 1 <br> ☐ 1 | ☐ 2 <br> ☐ 2 | |
| Wrist | flexion <br> extension | ☐ 0 <br> ☐ 0 | ☐ 1 <br> ☐ 1 | ☐ 2 <br> ☐ 2 | |
| Fingers | flexion <br> extension | ☐ 0 <br> ☐ 0 | ☐ 1 <br> ☐ 1 | ☐ 2 <br> ☐ 2 | /24 |
| **TOTAL RANGE OF MOTION AND JOINT PAIN, UPPER LIMB** | | | | | /48 |

*Reference:* Fugl-Meyer, A.R., Jääskö, L., Leyman, I., Olsson, S., Steglind, S. (1975) The post-stroke hemiplegic patient. Scand J Rehab Med; 7:13-31

# ACTION RESEARCH ARM TEST

Patient:                                    Centre:

Examiner:                                   Date :

## A.    Subtest Grasp

|   |   | Evaluation | |
|---|---|---|---|
|   |   | Left | Right |
| 1 | Woodblock 10 cm <br> (If score = 3, total = 18 and go to Grip) | | |
| 2 | Woodblock 2.5 cm <br> (If score = 0, total = 0 and go to Grip) | | |
| 3 | Woodblock 5 cm | | |
| 4 | Woodblock 7.5 cm | | |
| 5 | Cricketball 7.5 cm diameter | | |
| 6 | Stone 10 x 2.5 x 1 cm | | |
| **SUBTOTAL** *Grasp* | | /18 | /18 |

## B.    Subtest Grip

|   |   | Evaluation | |
|---|---|---|---|
|   |   | Left | Right |
| 1 | Pour water from glass to glass <br> (pronation) <br> (If score = 3, total = 12 and go to Pinch) | | |
| 2 | Tube 2.25 cm <br> (If score = 0, total = 0 and go to Pinch) | | |
| 3 | Tube 1 cm | | |
| 4 | Washer over bolt | | |
| **SUBTOTAL** *Grip* | | /12 | /12 |

*From:* ARM Arm Rehabilitation Measurement, © Thomas Platz, 2005

## BOX AND BLOCK TEST

**Patient:**                                    **Centre:**

**Examiner:**                                  **Date :**

| | Left | Right |
|---|---|---|
| **Score** | | |

*Reference:* Mathiowetz, V., Volland, G., Kashman, N., Weber, K. (1985) Adult Norms for the Box and Block Test of manual dexterity. American Journal of Occupational Therapy; 39:386-391

*From:* ARM Arm Rehabilitation Measurement, © Thomas Platz, 2005

## C.  Subtest Pinch

|  |  | Evaluation | |
|---|---|---|---|
|  |  | **Left** | **Right** |
| 1 | Ball bearing, 6 mm, thumb and ring finger (If score = 3, total = 18 and go to Gross movement) |  |  |
| 2 | Marble, 1.5 cm, thumb and index finger (If score = 0, total = 0 and go to Gross movement) |  |  |
| 3 | Ball bearing thumb and middle finger |  |  |
| 4 | Ball bearing thumb and index finger |  |  |
| 5 | Marble thumb and ring finger |  |  |
| 6 | Marble thumb and middle finger |  |  |
| **SUBTOTAL** *Pinch* | | /18 | /18 |

## D.  Subtest Gross Movement

|  |  | Evaluation | |
|---|---|---|---|
|  |  | **Left** | **Right** |
| 1 | Place hand behind head (If score = 3, total = 9 and finish; if score = 0, total = 0 and finish) |  |  |
| 2 | Place hand on top of head |  |  |
| 3 | Hand to mouth |  |  |
| **SUBTOTAL** *Gross movement* | | /9 | /9 |

### Total score

| Total Score (all subtests) | /57 | /57 |
|---|---|---|

*Reference:* Lyle, R.C. (1981) A performance test for assessment of upper limb function in physical rehabilitation treatment and research. Int J Rehab Research; 4:483-492

*From:* ARM Arm Rehabilitation Measurement, © Thomas Platz, 2005